CRAZY! HOT!

and

LIVING ON THE EDGE!!

Shirley Harris-Slaughter

I dedicate this book to my husband, Langston, who was with me through the good, the bad, and the ugly, every step of the way. I could not have found healing without him by my side, supporting me and dealing with all of it.

Table of Contents

Introduction

I'm a healthy, happy, confident woman who just happens to be in what I consider the prime of my life – the sunny side of 70. Yes, you're reading this correctly, I am in my late 60s and proud. In fact, I feel vibrant! But… it wasn't always that way.

I used to have episodes of depression, punctuated by panic attacks. I'd get myself back together only to encounter another challenge. Everything began to spiral completely out of control around 1991, when my mother passed away. That was the most traumatic period of my life. I watched her go through surgery for cancer, and then five years later, go into a relapse. The doctors didn't have any answers for us. From my experience, they just did what doctors usually do — treat the patient with chemo without discussing viable solutions, or preventative measures for the future.

I took care of my mother from the beginning, when she first got the diagnosis, to the end when she lay dying in her bedroom, down the hall from where I slept. The stress of her ordeal took its toll on me, but I didn't actually get seriously ill until it was all over.

We got mother's hospital bill, and it added up to

about $200,000. For what? It would take a rocket scientist to understand the charges on that long statement. It was just too complicated.

I said to myself, "What my mother went through is unacceptable! There has to be a better way, and I'm going to find it!"

I had no idea at the time, what was lying in wait for me; lurking around the corner, waiting to grab hold and take me on a long, horrible ride. I would spend years grappling for solutions, and trying to find my way out of the bubbling caldron of health challenges that had ambushed me… and left me feeling helpless. From the emotional roller coaster called "crazy," to the dreaded "hot" flashes, and bouts of constantly "living on the edge," I couldn't predict what crisis was going to hit next. I tried to find answers while I was in a full blown medical upheaval, but no one gave me much to go on. To top it all off, I was suffering from early menopause because of a past bad decision to undergo a partial hysterectomy.

At the time, the doctors told me I would be fine. But in the end, I was anything but. It took years for me to put it all together – to make the connection between the surgery and the crisis that was unfolding in my life. With no facts and no real guidance, I was lost.

I didn't know where to turn. So, I did what I do best. I talked about it. Everywhere I went, I shared my story. Surprisingly, I discovered that other women were facing similar ordeals. As I listened to friends and acquaintances, and heard the stories that were so much like my own, I realized that I needed to write this book. There were so many individuals like me, searching for answers to their confusing health challenges. And, like me, they weren't getting anywhere. After a few nudges from well-meaning friends, I found the courage I needed to get moving on this project.

I am not a doctor, and do not present myself as one. I speak from my own experience only, and base my story and solutions solely on trial and error. From knowing my own body and what it requires for good health. I used my God-given gift of common sense to solve 99% of my health problems.

And that's the advice I'm now sharing with you. Read my story and learn from it. But also listen to your intuition. It is up to us to honor our bodies by heeding our inner voice, and filling our minds with knowledge about health and healing. When we do, we'll find more solutions in nature than we will at the bottom of a pill bottle.

Take my journey to heart and seek out the proper nutritional guidelines. Adopt an exercise regimen. Read, ask questions and become empowered. Reclaim your body and take over the reins of your destiny.

Shirley Harris-Slaughter

1

HEAL YOUR THOUGHTS, HEAL YOUR BODY

Stress is like rain. It starts with a trickle and before you know it, you're in the middle of a storm.

At least that's the way it was for me. As a young woman, my world was chaotic, and I didn't know what to do about it. The fact was, I wasn't handling my problems at all. They were handling me – in ways that I didn't expect. They were taking a toll on my health.

Stress is like that. As women, we try to be everything to everyone, and we sometimes hide our true feelings. In the process, we internalize the sadness, the fear, the worry, and the shame. It accumulates and surfaces as illness and depression.

Think about this for a minute...

CRAZY! HOT! and LIVING ON THE EDGE!

Most people who have dealt with migraine headaches will tell you that the minute they eliminate the root cause (a negative boss, a cheating boyfriend, or financial woes), the headaches clear up. This can be applied to most conditions. We can take control of our lives and reclaim our power by controlling our emotions, changing our attitudes, and making a few simple adjustments to our daily lives. Most of them are easy, convenient and free. They include:

- **Daily Walk through the park** -- This is not only good exercise. It can help the mind produce *endorphins*; a natural chemical that makes you feel content.

- **A Yoga class** -- About one hour of yoga once or twice a week helps the body release toxins. Yoga stretches help us release the anger, frustration, and sadness, that often gets trapped in our muscles. In addition, Yoga reduces symptoms of stress, and is particularly helpful for those coping with irregular heartbeat. If the Yoga poses seem intimidating at first, start slow and go at your own pace. You'll be surprised by how quickly your body adapts, and how much your flexibility improves.

- **Vitamin D** -- An afternoon soaking in the sunshine, gives the body a healthy dose of that all important and healing vitamin, known as

Vitamin D. This vitamin is critical for the development and maintenance of a strong immune system, along with strong bones and teeth. If you live in a cold climate, you can't always absorb vitamin D the traditional way -- directly from the sun -- but you can get it from natural orange juice, organic egg yolk, salmon, and other foods.

- **Positive Affirmations** -- The words you speak can help clear the mind and reduce stress. Simply make positive statements about yourself over and over. You can write them down, say them out loud, or repeat them quietly to yourself. Try this daily (about 25 times each morning and/or night) and you'll be surprised at how much better you feel.

- **The Right Veggies** -- Green, leafy vegetables are like an injection of medicine into the body. They are excellent for our blood because they fill our cells with *chlorophyll*, a vital nutrient for all life forms. Chlorophyll purifies the liver, strengthens the immune system, stimulates the brain, and lowers the risk of heart disease and cancer. It can be found in veggies with bright green pigments like kale, lettuce, wheat grass (best when juiced), spinach, mustard sprouts, broccoli, and even collard greens (the ones that aren't overcooked and saturated with pork).

You see, true power is in our own hands. The body is always trying to achieve perfect health, but we have to help it out by giving it proper nutrition, lots of rest, and a steady stream of good vibrations (meaning good thoughts). This is especially true when dealing with the stress referenced at the beginning of this chapter. The bottom line is that, you must deal with stress before it deals with you.

I found that out in 1974. At the time, I was having severe menstrual cramps, chronic female itching, and piercing headaches. I also had insomnia, and constant flashbacks. It was a period in my life that can best be described as a scene out of a horror movie. I realized over time that I was suffering from post-traumatic stress disorder (PTSD). I came to this conclusion after several years of suffering. You see, I would wake up suddenly in the middle of the night, with my heart racing. I was in a state of panic. It was as if something was pursuing me, and I was running like mad to get away. I was breathing rapidly, and was in a frame of mind that can only be described as sheer terror.

My bouts of anxiety began during my separation and eventual divorce from my first husband. We were only married three years, just long enough for me to get in, have a baby, and run for my life. From the beginning, it was a tumultuous relationship. He was verbally and physically abusive, self-destructive, an alcoholic, and a drug user. He also had no ambition, and I knew that if I didn't leave him, he would set a bad example for our son. But, just as I suspected, he fought against the separation. Why wouldn't he? I was a good Catholic girl with a good upbringing.

When I told him I was leaving, he vowed that he would never let me go. True to his word, he stalked me, showing up at my home, and appearing sometimes "out of the blue." During our separation, he carried out a campaign of phone harassment and threats. One day, he surprised me with a visit to the parking lot outside where I worked. On my way home, I was getting into the car when he jumped into the driver's side, pushed me over to the passenger seat, and took off. I was so stunned; all I could do was cry.

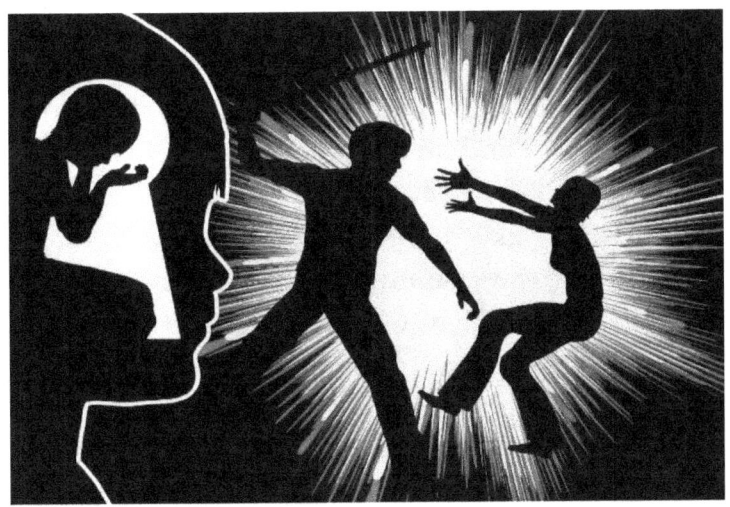

He took me to a cheap hotel somewhere in Detroit, tied my hands to the bed with two pieces of thick rope, and held me there overnight. I was distraught, crying, and hyperventilating. He threatened to harm me... to take me to Flat Rock where he was employed by Ford Motor Co. Despite my fear, I was able to muster up the courage to talk him down. I diffused the situation by telling him that if he let me go, from that point on, I would do anything he asked. Of course I was lying, but he was so irrational at the time. Eventually, he willingly drove me back home.

After that, I filed a personal protection order, and was never assaulted by him again. But, the ordeal was so terrifying it haunted me for quite a while, and I'm sure, it was the trigger for the PTSD and the Night Terrors. I don't know why, but it took me many years to figure this out.

I recall one night, while preparing my baby son for bed, I sat down and laid him on my chest to rock him to sleep. Suddenly, I started to feel this tightness in my chest. It felt like I was being squeezed, and it continually got worse until I was writhing in agony and pain. I had difficulty breathing. I kept gasping for air, but I just couldn't get enough in my lungs. My mother called for help, but when the police arrived and offered to take me down to Detroit Receiving Hospital, she exclaimed, "Over my dead body! You are not taking my daughter downtown!"

CRAZY! HOT! and LIVING ON THE EDGE!

At that time, Receiving Hospital had a reputation for admitting a lot of violent criminals and crime victims, and she didn't want me in that environment. So, the officers left. Fortunately, they returned, with the decision to take me somewhere closer to home. We rode to Mt. Carmel Mercy Hospital aka Sinai-Grace Hospital, right in our neighborhood. The doctors went through the normal line of questioning, including personal inquiries about my marital status. When I told them I was separated from my husband, they looked at me with a sympathetic but knowing expression on their faces.

"OK," one of them said. "That explains it all."

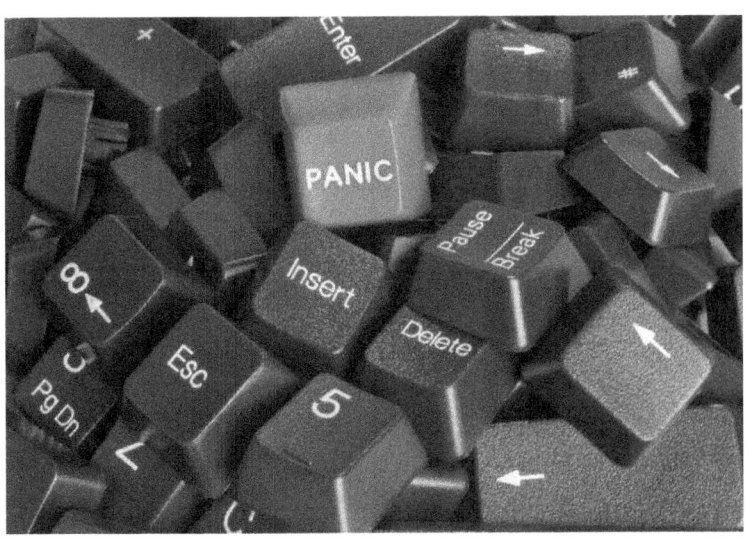

The doctors went on to explain that cases such as mine – a young woman having sudden episodes of anxiety – were all too common. They called them panic attacks. They prescribed Valium which helped control the symptoms.

That night, I learned what stress can do. It can practically kill you.

Around that time, I began to feel despondent. I was so ashamed of my life, and the bad choices I had made. I also continued to experience more episodes. Then, one day, my mother looked at me and said, "Maybe you need to go back to your husband."

Don't get me wrong. It's not that my mother didn't understand why I filed for a divorce. She supported me in every way possible. However, she was worried about my health, and believed that I would feel better if I worked out the problems in my relationship.

I remember saying, "No, mom, just let me get through this. I'll get over it no matter what it takes!" I may have been sick and filled with despair, but I refused to go back to him.

My doctor referred me to a psychologist for several sessions. During my first session, the psychologist just stared at me. Beyond introducing himself, he literally didn't open his mouth to say much of anything. We sat there for an hour staring at each other. It became very uncomfortable for me. Finally, I said, "It's been nice knowing you, but I think I can handle this on my own. I'll call you if I need you in the future."

And I thought I was crazy!

I did eventually get through it. But at the back of mind, I was always worried and afraid that I would have another attack. It was frightening.

Meanwhile, a barrage of new health issues began to flow into my life. One of the biggest ones was *Diverticulosis*. Attacks were often triggered by eating peanuts or popcorn with kernels in them. Diverticulosis is identified by pockets in the colon walls where certain kinds of foods can become trapped, causing excruciating pain in the lower left side. That is what I began to experience.

My doctor told me that it's caused by the typical low-fiber Western diet. And all that time, I thought I was eating well. What a joke! As if the misery in my life wasn't enough, I now had to contend with the fact that my diet was unhealthy. True, I used to eat the occasional hamburger and fries, but my (present) husband was a good cook, so I thought his meals were nutritious. I used to love eating his scrumptious southern fried chicken and delicious pork steak. Imagine my disappointment when I learned that those foods were the first things that had to go.

But I was determined to change my eating habits and improve my health. I began buying organic veggies and fresh organic fruit whenever I could. This helped somewhat. But, I was still in a rut. I was stuck in what a prominent minister and author, the Rev. Joyce Meyers, calls "stinking thinking." My mind was still fixated on everything that had gone wrong. I later learned that even a healthy diet wouldn't put me on the road to wellbeing and vitality, if I couldn't unplug my mind from all the negativity of my past. The stress had to be eliminated! Whenever I got sick or just felt under the weather, stress was always the culprit. But, my problems continued to mount. Whenever I tried to start an exercise program, I would get sidetracked by an illness that wouldn't leave me with much strength to do anything strenuous.

If I planned to go out for lunch with an acquaintance, I would suddenly have to cancel because my health would fail me yet again. I couldn't handle irritations in my everyday life very well, and that would cause my stress level to rise. I became bitchy. It got to the point where I couldn't stand myself, and I knew I was turning off everyone around me. But, I was powerless to stop it. It felt like I was losing my mind.

Did I want to be happy? Yes! I just didn't know how. My emotions were way out of control, and despair was ruling my world. I was desperate to understand all this craziness, and do something about it.

As I said earlier, I'm much more upbeat these days.

I've made a lot of mistakes along the way, and I must admit, the journey is ongoing. But, I'm pleased to be able to boast about my health instead of complaining about my illnesses. In the next few chapters, I'll do just that. I'll point out my missteps – the landmines you should avoid! Then, I'll lead you along an exciting path filled with alternative medical practices, delicious, natural food choices and – at long last – days and nights of pure peace.

2

ANGELS IN THE MIDST

We've all heard, and perhaps, sung a few lines from Beyoncé's catchy song, "Halo." But that song has an even more special meaning than most of us probably realize. In the lyrics, there's mention of walls "tumbling down." There's also a line that suggests, "It's like I've been awakened." Well, that's a crucial message. Basically, we all have to break down walls that have been erected by a society that encourages us to drink soda, eat salty, fatty snacks, and devour so much red meat we might as well be lions on the prowl.

Those walls that surround us include advertisements on TV, flashy messages on the Internet, and even on billboards and magazines. We live in a world where the burger is king, and starchy French fries are a staple food. Those walls had to come down.

When it does, we will feel as the song suggests -- like we have "awakened." Seriously, that's how I feel now when I look back and recall the way I used to eat, and the attitudes I used to nourish. I had left the bad marriage behind me, but not the resentment. I had moved on to a new life, but the old life was still haunting me, and festering inside of me. As a result, my life had become a dark, winding highway filled with potholes and speed bumps.

What's worse, I couldn't find an exit ramp. This led to one harrowing experience after another. For starters, I was not taking my anxiety medications correctly. Valium is a powerful narcotic, and should not be mixed with alcohol. I admit, I had been warned of this. But the doctor had such a heavy accent that I hadn't understood a word she said. I missed the message -- a misunderstanding that could have cost me my life!

One night, while out bowling with friends, I sat at the bar to sip on an alcoholic beverage. After about an hour, my head crashed to the counter, and a couple of the guys there had to help me home. I didn't know what was happening to me, but I knew it was bad. One of the guys had to drive my car, while I rode with the other. I was blessed to be in the hands of good people. They took care of me, and got me home safely. I never made that mistake again.

CRAZY! HOT! and LIVING ON THE EDGE!

Unbelievably, on every step of my harrowing journey, I met angels along the way who helped me either get through a bad situation, or rebuild my fragile self-esteem. These "angels" always seemed to be male. I even received a marriage proposal from a blind date. Talk about seeing "halos!" The guy who tried to make me his wife was like an angel in the sense that he helped me rebuild my self-esteem. He was educated, good-looking, and had his own radio show on Sundays. But, that's another story. The point is, my self-esteem had taken a nosedive during the marriage. The kindness and attention I received from that man during our blind date, helped restore some of my confidence.

I also had the comfort and support of a number of female friends. As I rebuilt my sense of self, and struggled to regain my inner strength, it seemed as if there was always a special girlfriend around, giving me advice, or simply listening when I needed to talk. I thought of them as angels then, and I still see them that way to this day.

Along the way, I met and married again, and my new husband turned out to be a terrific guy. He's a prime example of the notion that you can actually meet someone who "can love all the broken pieces back together." My mother was quite pleased and she told him so. She looked at him and said, "Now, I don't have to worry about my daughter anymore. It's on you."

She meant that in a good way. With my husband Langston's love, patience, and support, I calmed down and made it through the night terrors. He would hold me in his arms until I settled down. Over time, my heart stopped racing out of control, and eventually, the panic attacks disappeared.

Even though that traumatic part of my life was over, the damage was done. I still found myself mired in one health problem after another. And then, my mother passed away... and that sent me over the edge. After we buried her, my health spiraled out of control.

Just remember this: Whatever you do in your youth will either reward you as you age, or come back to haunt you in ways you never dreamed of -- especially if you're a woman! Add bad relationship choices to that mix, and you have a recipe for disaster. And disaster is what happened to me.

I cannot tell you the number of women I have talked to over the years, who were silently suffering from one problem after another. I'm talking about young women, too. I constantly share what I'm doing to help myself, and there never seemed to be a shortage of ears eager to listen. There is definitely a void in the medical information pipeline. And I can't believe the number of young women I met who had serious health issues, including early menopausal symptoms and weak bones.

Other examples include: Celiac Disease (a sensitivity to wheat products), Leaky Gut Syndrome (when particles of food actually leak out of the colon and into the bloodstream), and Irritable Bowel Syndrome (IBS), a disease that would later surface in my colon. Leaky Gut, Celiac and IBS all involve irritation of the colon, leading to either diarrhea, constipation, gas and other discomforts. Until I dealt with IBS, I had never heard of any of these ailments. I realized that there were a number of illnesses that seemed to be impacting so many individuals.

My question is why?

Based on my research, the reasons vary:

- Not enough fiber in the average American diet (Fast foods, junk foods & processed foods)

- Soda and other carbonated, sugar-laden beverages

- GMO's (genetically modified food)

- Foods saturated in sodium, harmful dyes, and other chemicals

- Stress

Stress may be last on the list, but it's actually one of the chief culprits. Our hectic, fast-paced society, places constant demands on us to achieve, get things done, shop till we drop, and juggle parenting with job responsibilities. We're living in a high-tech world, and our diets are crammed with processed foods saturated with chemical additives. In our attempts to be superwomen, we're looking for convenience – quick money, quick carry-outs, and easy-to-prepare, quick family meals. And we're paying a high price for our lifestyle.

My husband used to make me relax for fifteen minutes when I came home from work. After fighting rush-hour traffic while traveling from downtown Detroit, I was usually in anger mode. So, those precious minutes helped me so much.

Too bad, I didn't apply those same principles in my later years, especially after my mother passed away. Her death put me in a new and different kind of stress mode. I couldn't relax in my home for the longest time, because that is where she died. I wasn't eating or sleeping well, and my health started to spin out of control. It happened before I became aware of it.

Family pressures placed a strain on me and my husband, especially when it came to our children – his and mine. Langston is easygoing, and nothing seemed to get to him. On the other hand, I don't deal very well with family drama. It caused me to lose sleep, sometimes keeping me awake all night, stressing over some issue. And, of course, that would wreak havoc on my physical health.

Then, like most people, I went to doctors and expected them to fix it. The problem was that, most of the medical profession is trained to apply a band aid, not a cure. And most doctors are conditioned to respond to an illness after it's already raging in your body, rather than teaching us what to do to prevent it in the first place.

Here's a news flash: Doctors are not as perfect as we think they are, whether male or female. As women, we tend to think that female doctors know more about what's going on with our bodies, because we share the same gender. Ladies, I hate to break it to you, but most women doctors don't know either, at least that theory played out in my personal experience. And so, I found myself sharing information, or telling folks who to go see. I kept saying that I needed to write this stuff down, and one day share it. I wanted people to know there actually is a natural road back to good health.

Everything I have learned has been the result of mistakes made and learning from them, and using the common sense that God has bestowed upon me, and each and every one of you. It is up to you to use it. When you do, you will get help along the way, from unexpected sources, and even from angels walking among us.

3

A MEDICAL CRISIS

I was working on a temporary job assignment for a large corporation when the worst thing that could happen did! After finishing my lunch in the building cafeteria on the ground floor with my colleagues, I stood up, and all of a sudden, I had a terrible cramp in my lower abdomen. I had to get to the restroom fast, but couldn't move. I was losing muscle control of my bowels! I slowly worked my way out of the cafeteria, leaning against the wall just outside the door in order to brace myself. I took deep breaths and prayed, then slowly, steadily, I eased my way to the nearest restroom. It was just horrible and humiliating.

After a few more episodes like this, I made an appointment to see a gastroenterologist (a specialist in digestive disorders) to find out what was going on. The procedure is called a Colonoscopy. It was performed in the specialist's office around 1995.

I was instructed to do an enema at home, so that my colon was empty and cleansed before the procedure could be done. Imagine my surprise, on my appointment day, when I realized that they weren't prepared for me. I was left sitting in the waiting room instead of being taken to a room to get ready for the procedure. So, the doctor was upset that his staff didn't seem to know what to do when my time came to see him. I couldn't understand it, and neither could the doctor.

I was not given anesthesia, and so the procedure itself was very painful. They had to insert a tube into the rectum to examine the condition of the colon. My body was trying to push out the offending object, and doing it violently. In hindsight, I never should have had it done while awake. I never forgot this because I remember being in so much pain. I didn't feel that the medical team was taking good care of me.

Finally, I got a diagnosis: Irritable Bowel Syndrome -- also known as IBS! After suffering through bouts of digestive distress, it all came down to these three letters! The doctor told me that I would have to live with it. He prescribed medicine to control the spasms in my colon, but they had to be taken a half hour before each meal. Imagine forgetting to take a pill, and your family sits down to eat, and then you remember you have to take it and cannot enjoy the meal with them because you have to wait for half an hour? Did you honestly think that I would go through that forever? Not on your life!

I recall my very first colonoscopy. It was done in a specialist's office in the mid-eighties under anesthesia. When I woke up, the diagnosis was revealed – Diverticulosis! There was no pain and I woke up feeling relaxed, knowing that this medical doctor took extra care of my well-being.

I had never heard of Diverticulosis. Couple that with IBS, and you have a recipe for disaster. I wasn't able to travel with my husband at all, with this condition. The loss of the ability to control your bodily functions takes away any semblance of freedom you have in life. This affliction starts to control you, and there is nothing you can do about it but find the nearest restroom if the urge hits. The last place you'd want to be is on a plane; or anyplace, for that matter, that did not have a restroom nearby. It was an awful way to live, and so I stayed home and became a recluse.

Living a carefree life was simply impossible. I had to find my way out of that nightmare, which is what my life had become. My mother used to say that "God helps those who help themselves." With those words in mind, I made myself a promise that I would find a solution to my problems… no matter what it took. That night, I threw all the pills in the wastebasket. I was serious! I was not going to live like that.

It's amazing how quickly solutions can come. That same night on Diane Sawyer's evening broadcast, I discovered Dr. Andrew Weil, a medically licensed holistic doctor who had made the decision to do more with medicine than just prescribe pills. He sounded like my kind of doctor. I went to my local bookstore, The Book Beat, to buy his book, *Spontaneous Healing* - and it put me on a path to a much healthier lifestyle.

I was delighted by the natural steps it listed as guidelines for getting on the right track to good health. Before reading *Spontaneous Healing*, I was clueless. After reading it, I felt motivated and empowered. Dr. Weil taught me how to let go of old, self-defeating habits, and establish a new set of daily rituals. At first, I was a little intimidated because I wasn't sure I could let go of the old routines, and implement such drastic new ones. But, I was inspired by the examples in his book, of people who had healed themselves naturally. I told myself that if they could do it, then I could too.

I also knew that I had to dig myself out of the prison I found myself in – a deep, dark hovel of misery, confusion, and chronic tummy aches. I had to escape. The interesting thing was that, once I embraced the alternatives in the book, I found that they weren't as hard as I had thought. Weill's suggestions included a number of positive, helpful practices. Some I followed to the letter, but others simply weren't for me. However, I made at least six adjustments to my routine that impacted me so positively, that I continue to follow them to this day. They are:

1. Getting rid of my electronic alarm clock, and going back to a simple wind up clock. This was an important decision, because it's something that never would have crossed my mind to do. It turned out to make a major difference in the way I coped. You see, it's all part of living in harmony with natural law. Let's face it, we use so many digital gadgets, that all of us are steeped in low radiation on a daily basis. Switching back to my old tick-tock alarm clock was one small step, but I actually slept better at night, and had more peace of mind during the day.

2. Not using the microwave oven (in my case I decreased the use).

3. Eating more vegetables and fruits all day, every day.

4. Homeopathic and naturopathic therapies.

5. Incorporating ginger (which has powerful healing properties) into many of my family's meals.

6. Breathing Exercises.

These new practices helped me a great deal, but my nightmare was far from over – not by any stretch of the imagination. Oh no! It was just beginning. But, I was planting my feet on a firmer, healthier foundation. These are prerequisites to good health. I was telling an acquaintance my story, and how out of disgust, I threw away the pills that controlled my spasms. He told me it was a good thing I did, because if I had stayed on those pills for a long period of time, it might have collapsed the muscles in my entire colon. Thank goodness I had sense enough to get off those, and many other pills that were prescribed for me over the course of my deteriorating condition.

I'm not touting this individual as a medical doctor. This conversation stood out in my memory as a stark reminder of the fact that far too many pills have far too many serious and dangerous side-effects, but they're perfectly legal to sell in this country. So much for looking out for the public's best interest. I have to look out for my health because I belong to that 1% who are susceptible to getting bad reactions from any drug they take. So, I have to be vigilant of what I am prescribed at all times, and from all sources.

I discovered that my pharmacist was also looking for other alternatives to western medicine. He said, "I don't do pills." Can you believe that? He was a pharmacist and even he refused to buy into what his own employer was selling to the general public! By that time, I had amassed quite a collection of pills and knew I had to stop the madness. I thought back to the promise I had made to myself years before, that I would not be one of those people with a counter full of prescription drugs that would force me to choose between a pill and eating a decent meal. I had seen too many seniors doing just that, and I thought it was absolutely shocking.

Shortly after discovering that my pharmacist was turning away from traditional medicine, I found out purely by accident, that my periodontist was going the alternative route, as well. I ran into him at a Whole Foods Market, which was my grocer of choice. That didn't necessarily mean that he was changing his way of life. But, the fact that he did this in the early 90s, a time when most people were not yet aware of natural alternatives, led me to this conclusion: While certain medical professionals were making a fortune off people like me, some of them were discovering ways to live without the dangerous medicines they were prescribing. I decided to pay attention and focus on what was really going on.

Speaking of periodontists, I stopped having to see mine after several years of treatment for a condition I developed in my early thirties -- Pyorrhea Aka Gingivitis or periodontal disease. The specialist performed oral surgery on me twice, cutting my gums, trying to stop the infection from spreading. When I made some changes in my lifestyle, the disease left me. I never had to go back to a specialist again. My gums are stronger than ever. I cannot pinpoint when the healing began, but noticing the gradual improvement, I thought it was a miracle. Incorporating lifestyle changes, diet, and getting nutrients into my system, all contributed to this dramatic healing. It was just so amazing!

I was on the lookout for a qualified medical practitioner who could treat me unconventionally. I was not having a lot of luck with conventional medicine. In the meantime, I started watching what went into my mouth which led me to The Good Food Company in Troy, Michigan. Later, I found Whole Foods and Natural Food Patch. These places gave me a choice of natural foods and supplements to ingest. I had to become pro-active in my quest for better health, and that included keeping a close watch on my diet.

You see, I suffered from food allergies too. You name it, and I had a reaction or some version of it. I was in that one percent that the doctors didn't know what to do with. I woke up one day and my skin had ruptured all over. My back was covered with eruptions, my front, arms and legs as well. I was scared because I didn't know what was happening. I was sent to an allergist and it was a nightmare trying to figure out why I was breaking out all over my body.

It turned out to be food allergies for sure. My body was no longer able to filter out all the poisons that had taken up residence in my body. I also developed an intolerance to fragrances from perfumes, aerosol sprays, cigarette smoke, and cleaning products. My lung capacity had diminished considerably, and I tired easily. Again, I had to figure out a solution all by myself, and that's where the discovery of colonics came to be so important to me on my journey to good health.

While going through this period, I couldn't keep anything on my stomach. I couldn't eat anything. I felt hungry all the time. I eventually came to the conclusion that there was a link between my consuming dairy products, and the digestive distress that was plaguing me. A diagnosis of 'lactose intolerance' only confirmed my suspicions. Looking back, I should have listened to the doctor who had cautioned me long ago to remove dairy products from my diet. The constant stomach sickness was a steep price to pay for not heeding the advice of an astute doctor. I love milk, ice cream, cheese, snacks with cheese, you name it. The thought of having to give up all my comfort foods was too overwhelming for me. Therefore, I continued to ignore the obvious signs and suggestions. I didn't give it any importance until a light bulb went off in my head and I said to myself, "You seriously need to leave dairy products alone. All of it!"

But I still couldn't quite accept it. I mulled it over in my mind, and tried to analyze the red flags I had ignored. As I looked back, I thought about the serious health issues that flared up after my mother passed away. I wondered if that was when the lactose intolerance took a turn for the worse.

Before the diagnosis of IBS, I documented everything I ate to understand why I could not keep my food down. The dietician suggested a diet full of wheat products. It wasn't until much later that I found out that wheat was the worst thing for me to eat. The dietician also added skim milk to the menu. That should have been left off, too. But the dietician didn't realize that I was lactose intolerant, and consequently, wasn't looking for it. I didn't find out until after the colonoscopy results came back. When I knew for sure that I had IBS, I realized that I needed to find a better solution. If I didn't, I would continue on the same path of literally dying a slow death. I desperately needed something to ease my IBS symptoms, as well as address the lactose problem. I was disillusioned and frustrated, but still frantically searching for answers.

My sister began worrying about me because I had developed dark circles under my eyes. My skin looked ashen all the time, and I looked old and terrible. My son said I looked like a raccoon. Although we laughed at that, it wasn't really funny. I knew that my situation was becoming gravely serious. I remember going to the supermarket and standing at the checkout counter when the cashier asked me, "Do you remember when bread was 5 cents a loaf?" I couldn't remember that far back. Boy, was I insulted. I thought to myself, "Did I look that old?"

I began to wonder if I really looked as bad as others thought. It wasn't until my neighbor stopped by to bring my mail (which had been delivered to her house accidentally), that I decided to really do something about all that was happening to me. Her comment that prompted this action was simple: "Are you OK?"

If you opened your door to someone, and the first thing out of their mouth is that question, then you know for sure, something isn't right. So, I started thinking, "I still can't digest my foods, so what can I do on my own to improve my situation?" Then I remembered the Juiceman Jr. Juicer that was stored in my basement, which had never been taken out of the box. I dashed downstairs, brought it up to the kitchen, opened it, and looked for the instructions and the recipe booklet that came with the unit. I went to The Good Foods Company and purchased organic vegetables, returned home, and started juicing. Hooray! I was finally going to get some nourishment.

The Good Food Co. in Troy, Michigan had an organic selection of groceries, and a restaurant housed in the store. Sadly, it is closed now. When Whole Foods moved into the same neighborhood, the competition proved too much for the smaller, older establishment. I started shopping at Whole Foods because it offered more variety of alternative food choices, including organic meats. The Good Food Co. never offered meat choices. If you have a partner in your life who will never be a vegetarian, it makes life easier when you have a wide range of food alternatives.

After I got on a juicing regimen, my niece came over one day and she immediately noticed a big difference in my appearance. She said, "Auntie, you look so vibrant!" Needless to say, I was shocked and happy to hear that I was looking much better. And all because I was drinking my fruits and vegetables. I was on to something… and it gave me hope.

The trick was using organic vegetables. Using pesticide-grown vegetables and fruits is a recipe for disaster. It can make you seriously ill, or make whatever illness you already have even worse. Apples are notorious for housing pesticides, so take care to only use organically grown ones. I am now a firm believer that if you use organically grown fruits and veggies, your health will improve by leaps and bounds. Vegetables are nature's miracle workers. It's just too bad this country uses too much pesticides on God's food supply. Such a shame! I'd heard that dandelion weeds are good for our health. Yet, we use poisons to eradicate them. We have so much more to learn about our planet, but first, we need to learn how to respect it.

I was talking to a friend of a friend once, who said she had tried juicing with disastrous results. She said that every time she juiced, she became ill. I asked her if she was using organic products, and she dismissed my question. Some people are not open to what you have to say, so they are not going to listen when you're trying to enlighten them.

Trust me when I say this:

The key to getting well is to have an open mind. Be willing to listen, no matter how farfetched the idea may sound to you.

Another myth we've been led to believe is that milk products are healthy. They are not! A booklet called "Don't Drink Your Milk" caught my attention one time, and so I purchased a copy. What stood out was the subtitle on the cover, "Milk is for Calves, not Humans." Among other things, the book explains that we are the only species on earth who drink another animal's milk as we age. After thinking it over, it didn't take long for me to agree with that analysis. It made a lot of sense.

Finally, something was working well for me, so I made it a permanent part of my health regimen. I vowed to never stop nourishing myself with organic produce and other alternative foods. I knew that improper eating habits would trigger an attack of my Diverticulitis.

Here's an example of what I was buying and preparing:

- Any and everything organic -- potatoes, vegetables, fruits
- Rice milk, almond milk, and other alternative milk products; or no milk
- A daily "Colon Tonic" – This involves juicing 6 carrots, one 3-inch wedge of green cabbage, and half an apple. Of course, all of the ingredients were organic!
- Apples and carrots for juicing, cabbage, spinach, almonds, grapes, bananas, strawberries, berries, lettuce & tomatoes for salads, hummus for spreads, broccoli, and squash for making stir fries. I juiced a handful of spinach and 6 carrots on a regular basis.
- When I had a bladder infection, instead of going to the doctor for an antibiotic, I would drink organic cranberry juice concentrate, adding water to decrease the strength. Cranberry juice -- also known as nature's miracle cure -- works like a charm every time. Antibiotics, on the other hand, wreaks havoc in the colon.
- Grain-fed beef and chicken. These are livestock that roamed freely and ate nourishing, toxin-free grain, as opposed to being cooped up in a

pen and stuffed with foods laced with antibiotics and other chemicals.

It was like the diet of Paradise. Every day, I ate a piece of toast using Alvarado St. Bakery bread with hummus, or an organic egg over easy, organic cereal, or oatmeal with almond milk. Lunch consisted of a fruit smoothie, or veggie wrap, or even a sandwich if I must. Dinner - meat and vegetables, or a veggie stir fry. It might sound complicated at first, but as you get used to preparing these types of meals, it's actually simple and easy to follow.

Just remember:

- Breakfast – Smoothie
- Lunch -- Salad and almonds, nuts for snack
- Dinner -- Stir fry with grain-fed meat or chicken & vegetables
- Snacks – Fruit smoothies; nuts

My husband ate what I ate with a few exceptions. Sweets, for instance, are his main vice, and he refused to let his cookies, pies, and cakes go. But, he was worried about my health, and wanted to do as much as he could to adjust and assist me -- from changing what we ate, to making adjustments to the household products we purchased.

I had started breaking out in hives and ruptures, and had extremely dry skin which would crack in specific places. In the early 90s, my husband and I addressed this problem by investing in a water softener from a company whose name escapes me now (they went out of business). Then, we contacted a company called Culligan. The company installed special filtration fixtures on the kitchen faucet and under the sink. This made it possible for the family to bathe in water free of fluoride, bleach, and other toxic chemicals. A reverse osmosis system was added for our drinking water, with its own little faucet installed. It has made a big difference. I drink lots of water now, and my skin is no longer dry.

Initially, I started out using Dove because it was the only soap that didn't irritate me. I try to avoid anything with fragrances since most of them caused minor skin eruptions, and some were causing me to have severe break outs. I began buying soaps from health stores such as Natural Patch, Whole Foods, and GNC. I even buy toiletries and toilet paper from places like Whole Foods. To this day, I don't use bleached toilet paper against my skin, and I can't tolerate the smell of perfume and hairspray. I would get a sore throat and a hoarse voice, and my nose gets stuffy like when you have a cold.

Inhaling cigarette smoke had me coughing up blood – once! Unfortunately, my husband is a smoker.

He had to do all of his smoking in the basement or outside in the sunroom.

I had to get away from bleaches and house sprays and deodorant sprays, and anything that caused me to react. I got better once I eliminated the offending products. I was able to breathe much easier.

Before long, I noticed a major change. As strange as it sounds, I can't even pinpoint when it happened. It's almost as if I just woke up one day and my allergies had subsided, the pain in my abdomen decreased, and I no longer had problems controlling my bowels. This all occurred as a result of the changes in my home environment, and my healthy food choices – especially when I eliminated dairy, and underwent colonics treatment.

Based on my body's reaction, it's obvious that the diarrhea that plagued me (one of the symptoms of IBS), was a direct result of my lactose intolerance. I remember eating macaroni and cheese one day and getting the runs immediately. Clearly, the adjustments in my diet and the elimination of milk helped me get my condition under control. (Around this time, I also added digestive aid enzymes to my diet regimen, but I'll talk more about that later.) The bottom line is that the IBS and Diverticulosis were almost gone. And the pill popping has stopped. Yes, I was free! Well, almost. I'd like to say that I rapidly joined the land of the happily and healthy ever after. But I still had a long way to go. There was a dark side to all of this and I was about to meet it head on.

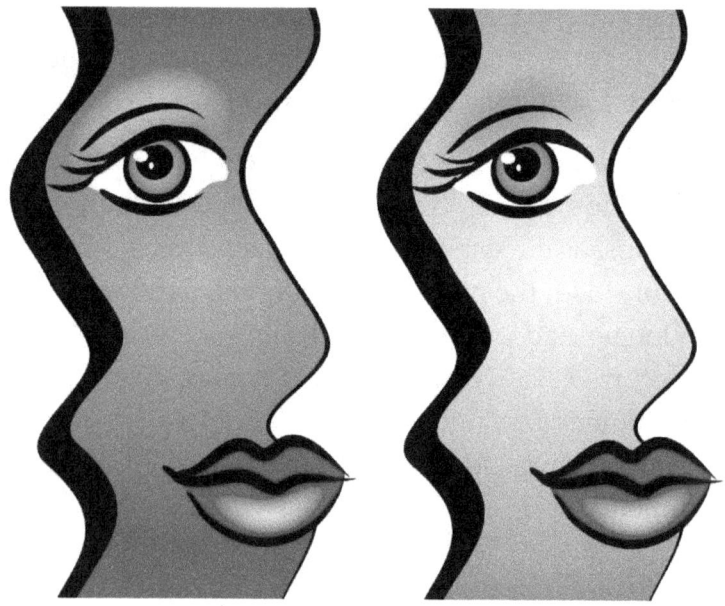

4

MEET THE DARK SIDE

You know that old saying, "If you don't use it—you lose it? Let me explain.

I had a partial hysterectomy. My ovaries were never surgically removed. It was during a laser surgical procedure in the 90s that the surgeon took the liberty of examining my ovaries, and informing me that they were gone. How could that be? I had a partial hysterectomy in the mid-70s which means they removed the uterus but my ovaries were left intact. So, I was stunned by this unexpected revelation. I went searching for my hospital records to prove that I did have ovaries! The proof was there! It was just so unbelievable to me. How could this have happened?

Well, as I looked back, I remembered that I once suffered from a fibroid tumor the size of an orange, and went to consult with several doctors on possible treatments. All of them said the same thing. That if I left it alone, it could become cancerous. The recommendation was to surgically remove the tumor or remove the uterus to prevent a reoccurrence. I opted to remove the uterus after a reassurance that I would have no more problems. Besides, I was suffering from severe cramps and heavy bleeding, and something needed to be done to fix those too, and fast!

So, over time, the ovaries had simply dissolved. This would explain why I had gone into full blown menopause. I was in my 40s, and every conceivable problem that could happen was manifesting itself. This was shocking to me. I had never heard of anything like this happening before, and there was no one I could talk to about it. That's when I came to that old saying, that if you don't use it… you will lose it.

The years went by. I started experiencing sudden weight gain, and so I made another appointment to visit my doctor. I had always been a very tiny woman, weighing in from a low of 98, and at 125 pounds at the highest, after giving birth. Yet, I looked at the scale one morning and it read 140 pounds! Wow! Most people look at 140 pounds and say, "What's wrong with 140 lbs.? That's not heavy." But for me and my tiny frame, it was too much too fast. I couldn't walk without a cane because my knees and feet hurt, and my ankles were swollen. I had developed arthritis in my hands and joints.

At that point, I decided to stop eating meat. Unfortunately, I then lost so much weight that my husband began to express extreme concern. I looked almost skeletal, and let me tell you... that was scary! The weight loss around my shoulders was the most pronounced. Once again, my friends and family began to notice, and ask if I was OK. A culmination of these events gave me a new respect for hormones. You don't miss them until they're gone. This was my introduction to the dark side.

Because of my depleted hormones, another challenge had swept into my life like a thief in the night. Hot Flashes. No, make that Extreme Hot Flashes! They're an intense sensation that grip women in their middle years, and makes them feel as if they're living in the bowels of a burning furnace. I'm not kidding; it's that bad. I'm sure a lot of women reading this can relate to what the doctor did next. She asked me to watch a video about menopause, then she gave me a well-known drug that begins with a P. That's right! She prescribed *Premarin*!

That's the solution I got for trying to get some relief – something to bring me back in balance from the menopausal symptoms and hot flashes that were ruling my life… ruining my life might be a better description.

I looked at the prescription and thought, "What the heck is that?"

The answer: Urine from a pregnant horse.

I was confused. Not knowing what else to do, I dutifully watched the tape from beginning to end. But, I didn't have a clue as to what I was supposed to learn. I feel it is noteworthy to emphasize that my doctor was a woman . . . and because she was a woman, I expected *more* from her. I thought a woman should have somewhat of an insight into what another woman goes through, since she has similar experiences as a female. No such luck! I was wrong in that assumption.

Contributing to my state of agitation about menopause was the fact that I felt like I did not have anyone to turn to for old-fashioned, woman to woman advice. My mother died before I could get answers from her, and my mother-in-law didn't have anything to offer when I consulted her. I was on my own.

The side effects from the oral prescription of Premarin gave me problems. Therefore, the doctor wrote another prescription --- for a patch. I thought that it would improve my condition, however, that was not the case… I started breaking out from the glue on the patch. So, I had no choice but to stop taking that as well.

Finally, the doctors could do nothing more for me, and I became sicker and sicker. The hot flashes got worse—leading to severe "night sweats." If I pulled the covers on, I had to take them off about 15 minutes to a half hour later. If I turned the heat down… my husband turned it up.

One time, I was in the bedroom fanning myself when my hubby approached me, and I said, "Honey, it feels like hot air is blowing all over me!" He laughed at the expression on my face, and this exchange lowered my stress level somewhat. Humor *does* have its rewards! I wanted that heat "off" and he was "freezing." And so it went like that for some time.

Another symptom I experienced with menopause was, my boobs actually started to drop – not sag. Gravity was working overtime with me. It was so painful that I wore a bra day and night to get relief! I said, "Oh my God, is this what getting old is about? I'm not having any of this!" Once again, I began to look for remedies on my own. The first step was to invest in more comfortable bras, because the ones with the wires were "killing me." *Comfort was what I needed… not style.*

Now, keep in mind, these annoying flashes were added to my already bizarre mix of health challenges. I was ready to scream. I came to the realization that the quality of my life had hit rock bottom. Oh, and did I mention that I had always suffered with migraine headaches? Well, now they were back too, along with occasional episodes of sinus headaches.

Frequent bouts of bronchitis also had me running to the doctor's office on a regular basis, getting prescribed antibiotics, which I later learned only added to my failing digestive health. It got so bad that I started developing bad reactions to any and all kinds of drugs, especially antibiotics. I began writing down my reactions to these drugs to keep track. There were no other options out there. It was all very frightening. I was in the midst of a medical crisis!

I started tying my migraines in with hormonal changes. It took me my entire life to figure this one out. As I looked back, I recalled that my first attack occurred at the age of 16 when I went through puberty. I was sitting in study hall. All of a sudden, I saw these spots blocking my vision which got bigger and bigger, with an aura surrounding them that obstructed my peripheral vision. When it finally disappeared, I was left with a horrible headache on the right side of my temple. It was so bad, I had to lay my head down and close my eyes. I was sitting next to the window with the sun shining bright on me. I was to learn later on… that was the worst place to be.

Another lesson learned: It's better to be in a dark room away from any kind of light when an attack comes on. I told my mother about this experience, and she had no idea what was wrong with me. She took me to the doctor and I was told I would have to live with it. Throughout my teenage and young adult years, I suffered in silence and handled it as best as I could.

The migraines definitely limited the quality of my life, and my health became very fragile. I remember once at a company Christmas party, I consumed alcohol and became quite ill. I then suffered a migraine and had to retreat to the restroom and then home. I was taking birth control pills, and knew that I shouldn't have. The warning label had clearly stated that if you suffer from migraines, you should not take contraceptives. In order to avoid pregnancy, I took the risk anyway.

But there was a surprising side effect to this. Usually, I suffered from mood swings, severe cramps, and heavy bleeding during my cycle. Suddenly, there were no more bad cramps and no more heavy menstrual cycles. I was happy that I could function normally again, and would be able to stop missing work because of these "problems." The suffering was over. So, I rationalized that it all had something to do with hormonal imbalance. The birth control pill is a hormone. Most women I knew seemed to suffer from cramps (some more severe than others) and mood swings. Seems like everybody I ran into had the problem.

Thinking back, I also remember that whenever it was that time of the month, I would get so emotional that I would cry at the drop of a hat. If I felt someone talking to me the wrong way, I took it so seriously. And wouldn't you know it... every time I planned on going anywhere, it just happened to be that time of the month.

Years ago, my girlfriends and I were invited up to Western Michigan University. I was out of high school and was already working. I was still single and hadn't yet experienced what life was all about. In other words, I was naive. There were ten of us, and we were going to meet ten guys. I was so excited! The cutest one picked me out, but I later blew it. We danced that night and went out for drinks. My girlfriends and I swore we wouldn't tell a soul that we ended up in a dorm room with several guys (all friends, of course). The girls shared a mattress and the guys had the box springs. It was hilarious, now that I think about it. We were so young and innocent that we thought what we were doing was a crime, and promised each other we wouldn't tell a soul. Those days are long gone.

But, back to my point.

The next morning my girlfriend said, "Cry!" and I began crying hysterically for no apparent reason. She was only teasing because she'd noticed how distressed I looked, and wanted to "throw salt on the wound." Talk about crazy and living on the edge. I was the epitome of crazy. I was just not emotionally prepared to handle what was really only humor.

I went into the bathroom so my cute new friend wouldn't see me that way. I stayed in that bathroom for what seemed like forever, and when I finally came out, my eyes were bloodshot. I avoided him (I don't even remember his name now). I was too ashamed of my behavior to even look him in the eye. I thought I was losing my mind, but I now attribute my behavior to the raging hormones that always flared up during my monthly cycle. We left the university and returned to our everyday lives. I never saw the guy again. But the hormonal episodes had become a significant part of my life, and nearly every month, I experienced strange mood swings or some other health issue.

Another time, I remember babysitting for a parish member's four young children. I was standing in their kitchen, and for no good reason at all, I reached for a wound-up clock on the kitchen counter and put it up close to my left ear. Maybe I was bored and had nothing better to do. I was alarmed that I could not hear the tick! So, I moved it to my right ear and could hear the ticking loud and clear. I immediately called my mother. She took me to the doctor where I was diagnosed with a wax buildup so severe, that it would take several visits to get it all out. With the wax dilemma behind me, a new problem came in the form of loud, sudden noises. If a door slammed shut, it sounded like thunder, which startled me. It was almost as if I had post-traumatic stress syndrome. I was jumpy and on-edge all the time, trying to re-adjust to having a clean ear.

Most of my young life, I used my right ear to compensate for not being able to hear out of my left. I would fall asleep, ensuring I was not consciously sleeping on my 'good' ear. I used to pretend I could hear when someone whispered into my bad ear, but I always wondered why I couldn't hear them. It never occurred to me that I had a problem, until that ticking clock forced me to recognize it.

After the discovery and initial treatment, the buildup kept returning over and over again. I spent years trying to control it. Eventually, I was to learn what had caused such a severe wax build-up, and how to prevent it from re-occurring.

This may have been the first time a medical doctor told me to eliminate dairy products from my diet. I was still young and stubborn. I guess I wasn't ready to make a drastic change back then. So, I didn't heed that advice right away. I was also told to eliminate flour products, as in breads and all the other foods I loved. That was just too much to ask! The "Bread of Life" is a term used in religious gospels, so how could I be told to just give it up? Or was that just a metaphor for spiritual food?

Now, as an adult, I was finally getting the point. I began to realize that hormonal imbalances had actually reached epidemic proportions in this country. So I asked myself… why? Why was I so overwhelmed by hormonal problems, and why was I seeing so many people suffer from this affliction? And why did the Pill stop mine?

Now, I am not a doctor but I can speak from my own truths. I sincerely believe that hormonal problems are, indeed, being aggravated by our environment. Although I have no hard data, I have read a number of studies that blame some of our hormonal issues on plastic. Yes, you read that right. Plastic -- that synthesized material that is so prevalent in our society – has been noted for, among other things, revving up the hormones in women and girls. In fact, there is a strong suspicion that plastic is responsible for inducing premature puberty. American girls are entering puberty earlier than their foreign counterparts. Some of them (particularly African American girls) have been known to develop breasts and start their periods as early as 9 and 10 years of age. This used to be the exception.

Plastic isn't the only villain. I've seen young girls maturing at a rapid rate, and I've been told that it's coming from the hormones put in dairy animals that end up in the milk supply and other forms of dairy products. Children are eating whatever that animal was fed. These young girls have bodies of mature women and baby faces. It was odd and alarming to see. Fortunately, I don't see too much of that nowadays.

Chicken is another source. Unless they're free range, chances are, they were injected with hormones to fatten them up for quick sales and higher prices. Typically, the hormones are pumped into the factory farmed chickens stuffed into tiny cages. This is leading to rampant obesity and also causing widespread hormonal issues. In our country, everything is about money, and the powers that be don't seem to care who gets affected.

I know I'm making some strong claims, but the evidence is everywhere. Besides, this is the truth I was living with as I dealt with everything from premenstrual syndrome to searing headaches. Over time, the headaches started coming more frequently, sometimes two and three times a day. Headaches that frequent were alarming to me. Then, I met a wonderful doctor who suggested I get off birth control. This may not sound believable, but for several office visits, this doctor seated me in a quiet, dark room, with only the sound of soft music playing, and I never suffered another migraine headache again. He was a miracle worker, and I will always be grateful to him for placing me on the path to a headache-free life. But, I wasn't out of the woods just yet.

I was diagnosed with osteoporosis in the lower spine and had actually started developing a hump in my back. I went to a chiropractor who used natural approaches which actually removed the hump.

However, an MRI confirmed that my bones were thinning. I was frightened out of my wits.

Then, I remembered my mother's favorite scripture: "God helps those who help themselves." It was 2001 and I had come a long way – but not far enough. Langston was so worried about me that he stopped eating the way he should, even though he loves to cook. I was sick and he was concentrating his efforts on helping me get well and was neglecting himself. I couldn't travel because my health was just too fragile. I couldn't help my husband, until I was able to help myself. So, I kept on with the juicing which literally saved my life, and kept searching for a solution to my hormonal deficiencies.

They say seek and you shall find, and I did! I picked up a copy of Suzanne Somers book, "The Sexy Years." That book was magic. I read her story and looked to the back of the book for references. I wanted to find a doctor near me who could administer the Bio-Identical Hormone Therapy that got my attention. I had never heard of it, but I looked at Suzanne, observed how beautiful she was, and figured... why not try it? I found a doctor online who had an office here in my hometown. It was about 20 miles away, but I didn't care. I would do whatever it took to get well.

I met Dr. Pamela Smith around 2002. It took me a long time to find her. My problems had actually started when I had that partial hysterectomy in my early thirties. That was too young to have menopausal problems. A conventional doctor once said I had a fibroid tumor, and I would need to have a D&C which stands for a *dilation and curettage*. It's a procedure that involves having the lower part of the uterus dilated, in order to scrape abnormal tissues from the uterine lining. According to this particular doctor, fibroid tumors are prevalent among young black women.

And I said, "And????"

Needless to say, there were no answers forthcoming from him as to why this was so, and no solutions as to what to do about it. I was visibly upset that he could tell me that and yet offer nothing except a suggestion to have surgery if the tumor came back.

Well… it did, and it grew back to the size of an orange! I was scared and tried to seek a second opinion. Stupid me! I was going to the same type of doctors who spewed out the same solutions. Get surgery to remove the tumor, or you may get cancer if it comes back. I didn't know anything about alternative medicine, so I opted for the surgery, and that is how I eventually went into early menopause. They took the uterus and left the ovaries, but it didn't matter. I still suffered from having something taken out of my body that was supposed to be there.

I felt uncomfortable all the time, and would become overheated if I got too excited or angry. I never knew what was happening until my issues were full blown. How did I know they were full blown? I stepped on the scales one morning, and my weight had shot up extremely high, literally overnight. At least it seemed that way. I sought another doctor to confirm what I already suspected. It was official. I was on menopause. My hormones were depleted. And so, I was forced into a long and difficult journey to find answers.

Hot flashes had come a little early for me even though the doctors told me I would be fine. I can't pinpoint when the flashes actually started. It was a slow process... very subtle, and I just thought I didn't feel well. But, I was too busy with my family and marriage to think about it. All I knew was that I was short-tempered, and that I cried at the simplest provocation. It got so bad that I couldn't stand myself, and I wondered how anyone around me could stand me. I didn't understand the changes I was going through.

Since I couldn't fathom what was happening to me, I had no clue as to how to cope with it. I now have a new respect for hormones after my experience, and how they can control every aspect of your life. Without the right hormonal balance, you will go into a tailspin. My body was completely out of balance because I was not producing any hormones... period!

In the midst of all that was going on with me, my newly discovered alternative doctor placed me on Bio-

Identical Hormone Therapy, and added some multivitamins and supplements to the mix, as she came to know more about me and my specific needs. That worked for me. I was getting a better handle on my health crisis with the new treatment I was receiving. My skin regained its radiant glow, my hair became strong and full. Oh, I forgot to mention that I had been losing my hair. Talk about vanity. I think that is what really made me spring into action. Losing my hair? Oh No. That was not working for me at all! Nor was the thinning of my lower spine. I was ready to do anything to keep those two things from happening.

One of my girlfriends from high school was diagnosed with stomach cancer. And she was a nurse for heaven's sake! I couldn't believe it! I went to see her and was shocked by her appearance. She could not eat, and there was nothing the doctors could do for her. She went home to starve and eventually die. It was a miserable way to go, and it shook me to the core. I caught up with one of our girlfriends during that fateful visit. That friend told me later on that she was telling anybody who would listen, that my hair was gorgeous and full and bouncy. She wanted to know what I was doing. We should have been talking about the demise of our dear friend, but evidently my appearance was a positive distraction. All I could do was thank God for helping me find answers. I wished my friend had found hers.

CRAZY! HOT! and LIVING ON THE EDGE!

These incidents happen to serve as a constant reminder of how precious our lives are, and how we must work diligently to preserve it and live each moment to the fullest.

Getting back to Dr. Pamela Smith -- she literally saved my life. I was put on hormone therapy and my circumstances changed completely. My breasts stopped hurting, and the hot flashes became mild and tolerable. Although, my body will never be the same, I began experiencing a new normal as my illnesses dissipated.

You have to be proactive in advocating for your health and wellbeing. If you don't, the conventional doctors won't do it, and you will be on your own or at their mercy. Mind you, patients who think for themselves are considered a nuisance by the medical establishment, which has to be in control at all times. But being difficult can bring big dividends. I decided to fight back.

This is my health we're talking about – not theirs!

5

THE HEALING MIRACLE

Detroit was once the home of a majestic, castle-like train station, with high-ceilings, cavernous hallways and ornate architecture. But this former treasure is now an abandoned, dilapidated mess. So, one day I gathered some participants to help clean up the littered field surrounding it. I had already started a movement to bring back the station and this was part of the process.

They say that when we dole out blessings, those blessings come back to us three-fold. Well, I have to admit, that's been my experience – especially that day at the train station.

I was pulling a clump of unsightly weeds that had

grown in the front of the building, and picking up debris, when someone approached and asked me why was I wearing a face mask. I told him that I was allergic to weeds, pollen, and any unusual smells in the air and the mask helped me to breathe better. He simply handed me a card so I could schedule an appointment for a reflexology treatment. I had never heard of reflexology, so I just stared at him and stuffed the card in my pocket. But he was friendly and seemed kind. So, I listened as he described the process. He explained that all the nerves in the body ends in the feet. These nerve endings in the feet are like pressure points that help reveal what's going on in the body. Simply by massaging or pressing these points, a trained practitioner can detect malfunctions in a person's body.

I was intrigued, but hesitant. A year later, I made an attempt to get in touch with this gentleman at the Detroit Wholistic Center and Wholistic Training Institute of Detroit. Unfortunately, he wasn't in the office when I called. However, the receptionist suggested that I make an appointment to visit the center, and have one of their health therapists perform a colonic.

"What is that?" I asked.

"It's a cleansing of the colon using purified water," she answered.

She went on to explain that a special device was

used to gently draw the waste out of the body. She encouraged me to come in to view their video tape on how the process worked. I must say I was very impressed and filled with hope. Although my diet and health were beginning to improve, I still needed further relief from my digestive ailments.

After scheduling an appointment with one of the therapists, I learned even more about juicing and eating organic fruits and vegetables. I also learned some very interesting facts about the colon. For instance:

- You can't be healthy if your colon isn't healthy. Millions of Americans are dealing with digestive problems -- chronic gas, irritable bowel syndrome, rectal and colon cancer - and yet, the state of the colon is given little attention.

- Everything we consume has the potential to do two things: It will either heal us or it will harm us. It all depends on the type of foods we choose.

- About 20 percent of Americans are dependent on laxatives.

- Constant use of laxatives can destroy the health of your colon.

- A clean colon is a healthy colon. A clogged colon leads to constipation and disease.

- Stomach pains, belching, bloating and

flatulence, and acid reflux, are signs of an irritated colon.

- The colon contains both good bacteria and bad bacteria. The good bacteria, which can be found in foods like kefir, yogurt, and certain veggies, helps the digestive system. Too much bad bacteria leads to poor health.

I listened with keen interest and absorbed knowledge I'd never heard before. I knew then why I had met the natural healer that day at the train station. I also realized that colonics could be the final frontier in my journey to good health.

During the first cleansing, I felt uncomfortable as all the poisons were slowly drained from my body. I had a headache and awful cramps. But when it was over, I felt so much better. I had two more appointments scheduled, and finished the entire process in three stages. But, I was still suffering from digestive issues and hadn't figured out yet how to address it.

Soon after, I discovered another step in the tummy healing process – Enzymes! Remember when I said I would get to this topic later? Well, here it is!

When I first heard about enzymes I didn't realize they were just what I needed, and so it took me a little longer to get it through my head that many of my digestive problems stemmed from lack of proper digestive enzymes (good bacteria). It had taken me quite a while to accept the idea that I could not tolerate dairy products. Now, I was finally ready to embrace additional changes, and take the necessary steps to get digestive aid enzymes into my system. With the juicing, the cleansing, and finally, enzyme replacement, I was starting to really heal!!

In addition to getting colonics at the Wholistic Center, Dr. Pamela Smith added Ortho Biotic enzymes to help with my digestion. If you can't digest your foods, your life is simply over. I was glad to be able to eat again and enjoy my meals. And the good thing about this therapy is that, she still sends me to the lab every six months to check my hormones, to catch anything else that may be out of order. She is a good anti-aging doctor who speaks all over the country, and has several clinics and affiliations around Michigan.

Her impact on my life has been tremendous, for my health and my appearance as well. I'm an author, and my sister, Connie, saw me in a video taken at a book event put on for me by the local library in my community. You see, you don't really notice how you look until someone tells you. She thought I was gorgeous. She lived in another state, so we don't get to see each other often. She looked at my face and hair, and asked for the name of my doctor. Naturally I said, "Dr. Smith, you'll love her."

I added: "Unfortunately, she needs to be

accredited to your insurance, otherwise you will have to pay out of pocket."

While paying out of pocket might be a problem to some, I didn't care. My attitude about money is this: "You can't take it with you." Besides, Dr. Smith gave me a quality of life I never would have had, and that's something you can't put a price on. As long as I have the means, I would pay anything for her healing services.

I will tell anybody that money is useless if you are too sick to enjoy it. Take that money and get your health back. Get creative with your financing. You can recover it once you are well enough to work. Wouldn't you get a loan to go on a trip? Yes, you would! Why? Because the bank will lend you the money. Treat your health with the same importance as a vacation, and you will get your health back.

It's not easy, but the rewards are great. I had no one to help me find my way out of my nightmare. But once I resolved to find some answers, a way always opened up. Someone was always there to point me in the right direction.

As a side bonus, the bone mass in my spine started to increase in density after I started the hormone therapy. I was overjoyed. It was a miracle! I reversed the bone loss and my hair came back full and healthy. I couldn't ask for anything more than that.

For that reason, I have very little patience for naysayers and others who try to knock alternative practices. One day, while sitting in a traditional doctor's office discussing my health, I mentioned that I had come across a holistic center that offered colonics. I told this doctor that colonics are a cleansing method for the colon. I also explained that "all illness begins in the colon."

Think about it . . . that's the organ that digests food, eliminates waste, and nourishes the cells, which is a tall order! And guess what? Sometimes it needs "cleaning out" just like a car engine. Anyway, my doctor said, "I have a problem with folks who practice medicine without a license, so I can't approve of what you are doing."

I said, "You doctors are licensed to kill."

He started looking at me a little closer. He had an unruly patient on his hands.

He assigned the dirty work to the office manager. While sitting in the waiting room, the manager informed me that the doctor could no longer help me, and that I should find someone else. I got away from him fast. He wasn't helping me find a solution to my problem, and I was glad to be rid of him. I have changed more doctors than I care to think about. I was doing whatever it took to get satisfaction for my primary care.

Although I still had a few bouts of diverticulitis, I knew what to do to heal myself so that I wouldn't have to take hard core drugs. Juicing is the spice of life, and cabbage is the vegetable that kills the infection that triggers those attacks; just like cranberry juice cures bladder infections. Nature has everything I need to cure most of my ailments. I just had to be willing to do the work.

Another thing I learned from all of this was that the use of antibiotics was one of the major causes of my digestive afflictions. If I had looked at the warnings, I would have known that. Like I said earlier, antibiotics promote an overgrowth of Candida, a bad bacterium. It takes over your digestive tract, and kills the good bacteria that assist in the digestive process.

Now, I'm pleased to say that the good and bad bacteria live in harmony with my colon – meaning the good bacteria had won the war. And while bacteria might sound like a disgusting topic, they're a worthwhile investment. Look for foods that are labeled probiotic, and buy probiotics in capsule form at any health food store and in certain drug stores. Probiotic vitamins deposits millions of live, friendly bacteria directly into your gut. Having a doctor help you choose the right enzymes for your particular needs is even better, and I would encourage you to do that, from my own personal experience.

You might think all of this is strange, but believe

CRAZY! HOT! and LIVING ON THE EDGE!

me, your stomach will thank you.

6

A YOUNG GIRL vs AN OLD GIRL

While waiting in the mall at a retail clothing store counter to pay for my purchases, I ran into a young girl about 19 or 20 years old, who had some serious health concerns. We started talking and she shared with me how afraid she was to leave her doctor, because she was taking so many pills for her ailments. I looked at her like she had lost her mind. When you are that afraid to let go of a doctor, you really have to be educated. Doctors are not gods. They can make many mistakes, and that is what I remember telling her. Go to a health store and read up on the ailments you have, and try to at least get the proper nourishment to help you while you look for a saner doctor.

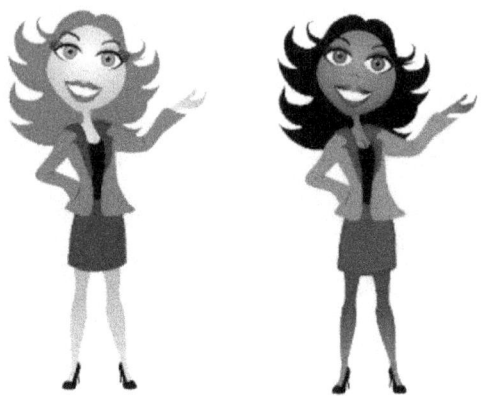

People are so hypnotized into believing everything their doctor tells them, that they don't use their God given common sense to think for themselves. The doctors today are not like the doctors in the old days. And when I say the old days, I can go all the way back to 400 B.C. and quote Hippocrates, the father of medicine. The Greek physician/philosopher once said:

"Let food be thy medicine and medicine be thy food."

That's wise advice that we all need to heed today. Instead of following the mindset of Hippocrates, present day doctors are trained to dispense drugs. They don't even study nutrition extensively. They get a small course in it, and a huge dose of knowledge that pills are the answer to everything. I do believe that some doctors are starting to catch on to the horrors of drugs just from listening to their patients. But not all are willing to admit it. Besides, pharmaceuticals are big business, and doctors are a part of that industry… unfortunately.

Amazingly, I've ran into many people who cannot handle the medication that's prescribed to them, and they have started looking for alternatives. My goal is to encourage more men and women, particularly young people, to check out these alternatives. If you don't, it can be pretty scary out there. You only get one body so why put it completely in the hands of someone who thinks a pill box is the only way for you to get well?

Listen to the doctor, then check out magazines, books, online publications and other resources for additional, back-up information. These are the tools you can use to empower yourself. If you're reading this, and thinking that there's not enough information available, you're wrong. It exists. You just have to dig for it.

Attend seminars at your local health food store. Whole Foods offers plenty of classes and workshops on the advantages of organic meals. Recently, I saw a posting about a session that discussed the healing properties of mushrooms. Detroit's Whole Foods recently offered a teaching class on plant-based foods. Go online to get upcoming events for your location. Keep your eyes and ears open, ask plenty of questions, and read as much as you can.

And when someone makes a suggestion, you don't have to accept it right away. But, whatever you do, please listen. When I met the young lady who was putting all of her faith in the medical establishment, I really wanted her to hear what I had to say and take it to heart. It could be that she heard me and that she is now doing her own exploration. Or it could be that she has no idea where to access the information she needs to heal. Again, the material is there if you hunt for it. This book is one example. It offers guidance on how to get on the road to good health, without being a slave to drugs.

I'm proof of that fact. My niece, whose journey is somewhat similar to mine, is another example. She could have easily fallen through the cracks if she had continued relying on the traditional health care industry. She suffered from weakening of the bones just like someone with osteoporosis. She also had depression, and was far too thin. Although it was threatening to damage her kidneys, she was popping Advil like candy. When I found out what was going on, I immediately directed her to get off of milk, and stop eating so much bread.

I introduced her to healthy supplements, and convinced her to eat organic fruits and veggies. To her surprise, she was able to regain her health and strength, just by changing the way she thought about her health. I helped her to realize that she was too young to be grappling with such severe health challenges.

But my niece and the other young women I encountered are not alone. I've met dozens of females in their 20s who are suffering with ailments so mysterious that I've never even heard of most of them. It is truly frightening. Women my age are dealing with their own ailments. In her late fifties, a good friend of mine was diagnosed with breast cancer and given a 40-50% chance of survival.

Well… guess what? Fifteen years later and she is still with us. I encouraged her to change her diet and adopt some of the practices I had tried. Fortunately, she listened. Her actions and prayers brought her through. I truly believe that her openness to receiving information is what saved her life. An open mind and a positive attitude are antidotes to disease, and are doorways to a brave new world.

And yet, so many of us cling to the side of the pool. We hang on, even when so-called remedies aren't working. We won't let go, although it's clear that our condition (whatever it is) has not taken a turn for the better. However, new ideas are like bursts of energy. They get us moving, and inevitably lead us to answers we may never have considered.

Here's another example of an idea that requires an open mind: Change your anti-perspirant.

CRAZY! HOT! and LIVING ON THE EDGE!

I have a theory that some might consider outrageous, but if you really think about what I'm about to say, you'll realize that many of them could be affecting women's health.

I came to this conclusion because I couldn't understand why there were so many breast cancer patients popping up. I decided to take a closer look at deodorants on the market that stop us from perspiring. That's when I discovered that there's an ingredient (aluminum chlorohydrate) that blocks perspiration, and can be found in most of the deodorants on the market.

This brings to mind a logical question: If you stop perspiring, then where are those poisons going to go? Back into the tissues of your body, under the armpits near your breasts. Trying to stop a natural process is probably not the wisest thing to do. There's an old commercial that states: "It's not nice to fool Mother Nature!" Maybe we need to take that to heart. Of course, we must have good hygienic practices, and certainly, there's nothing wrong with wanting to smell good. But, we don't have to use only antiperspirants to accomplish that goal. When I looked up that ingredient online, I discovered other people who think just like I do—using common sense solutions.

I go to the health store where I can find alternative choices. One of those choices is a citrus deodorant spritz called *Weleda*. Although I have to apply it several times a day, it's worth it. I've been doing this for approximately 25 years, and I think I have achieved the results I need to smell good and stay healthy at the same time. My friend who survived breast cancer has been following my advice and I have been open to her ideas as well. Her health is fragile, but she is still here.

And so am I.

Some people would call that a miracle.

7

DRUGS, DRUGS and MORE DRUGS

When I worked at a Catholic church on the east side of Detroit, Father Emiliano, an African priest out of Uganda was living in the rectory and attending Wayne State University. He developed cancer and was being returned to his home country. When the parish priest and I went to the drug store to pick up his medication, we couldn't believe our eyes. The store had a whole arsenal of pills rolled out for us. I was in a state of shock. I mean to tell you we could have started a drug store with the pills they gave us. It was criminal!

That poor man was too sick to take one, let alone try to follow a long list of directions. The irony is that Fr. Emiliano came from a culture that was accustomed to natural cures and remedies. In his homeland, people in villages often relied on herbs and spices as cures for what ails them. In some cases, they go into meditative trances and when they awaken, they are back to good health. They live in close harmony with nature, and many have a profound understanding of the habits of the wildlife in the forests that surround them. Once they leave the village, they take their knowledge and many of their ages-old traditions to the city. Depending on their tribe, (there are 80) Ugandans are a spiritual people, with a deeply abiding belief in God's supreme power to heal. They believe that God gave us vegetation with healing properties, and the inner wisdom to seek what we need. When they cook meat (beef or goat), they just cut it up into large pieces and cook everything in one big stew. Sometimes you don't know if you are eating meat, liver, intestines, stomach, tongue, or any other part of the animal because they waste nothing.

So, obviously, what was happening to Fr. Emiliano in this country was a tragedy. Yet, he was too ill and too sick to speak up for himself. I was upset at the neglect that this sick priest had to endure, and tried to help him as best I could.

Fr. Emiliano made it home and died shortly thereafter. It was so sad. He really didn't know how to take care of himself in the United States. In the Motherland, he, no doubt, would have eaten fresh, organic greens, finely chopped and mixed with onions.

In Uganda, fried plantains are popular, and ground nuts and lots of vegetables, yams and cassava, are staple foods. However, Father Emiliano was now immersed in our cultural practices, and didn't know how to reach out for help. Consequently, he didn't eat well. He went hungry many a day with no one knowing what was going on, including me. When the pastor of that church passed away, there was no one else to look after him. He was used to being cared for by the women back in his home country. It was the saddest thing I learned – and it was too late for me to help him.

This priest is just one example of what can happen to your health in a country that puts more importance on expedience, money, and greed, than it does on proper nutrition. My thoughts go back to this old lady I saw in the supermarket reaching for a gallon of milk. She was bent all the way over so badly that she could not stand straight up. I wanted to scream at her to put that milk down. Although I couldn't help her, she was a wakeup call for me. Just looking at her made me thank my lucky stars that it was not me.

But, just like I couldn't help Father Emiliano (although I tried), I knew I couldn't help this lady. There is no way she would have listened… and why should she? Everywhere she turns, there's another billboard displaying smiling people with milk mustaches above a caption that reads: "Got Milk?"

CRAZY! HOT! and LIVING ON THE EDGE!

Everywhere she turns, there's another radio ad featuring a gallon of creamy ice cream. And everywhere she turns, there's someone on TV boasting about how much better they felt after popping a tiny pill.

Have all those drug commercials ever caught your attention? Have you noticed all the side effects they tell you about -- including DEATH? Are they serious? Why do we allow this to bombard our TV screens?

We need to talk to our state representatives and declare war on the drug industry. Of course, it would take another book to discuss the corruption of the pharmaceutical industry, and try to explain the power this multi-billion-dollar industry has over Congress. They make money when we are sick. Just in case you didn't get that, I will repeat it. The pharmaceutical industry thrives when large groups of individuals are not well. It is in their best interest. They know there is a segment of the population that wholeheartedly believes the stuff they advertise. That segment trusts them -- like that young woman I talked about who couldn't wean herself away from her doctor's pills.

This has not always been the case. Back in our grandma and great grandma's era, it wasn't unusual to be told to drink freshly squeezed potato juice for heartburn or boil a potato, mash it, wrap it in cotton, and apply it against your skin to heal a sore throat. Castor oil and cod liver oil were like obsessions. No one liked it, but you better believe, it kept you from getting ill. And, when you do get sick, your grandma or one of your great aunts would give you an enema to clean you out. After that, you were fine.

Hospitals and doctors didn't oversee the health of our grandparents and great grandparents – especially not the ones who were still living on a plot of land. If they were in the Deep South and living on a farm, the nearest doctor's office was too far away. So, they didn't depend on pills. They weren't drowning their taste buds with salt and sugar either. They breathed fresh air, drank fresh water and often, ate food that they had grown. Oh, if only we could go back to those days.

Based on what's going on, it wouldn't be a bad idea. Currently, a company known as Monsanto is producing genetically modified seeds, and trying to gain control of farms around the country and the world. Monsanto -- which is already guilty of controlling and genetically modifying much of the corn, zucchini and soybean crops in the United States -- creates seeds that contain pesticides within them. This is a problem for obvious reasons. It means there's no need to bother washing pesticides off of the veggies and fruit you eat. You can't! If it's a GMO product, the pesticide is already inside of the produce and can't be eliminated. It also means that, with every bite you take, you're devouring chemicals. There are pros and cons to this argument. But, there is a concern about the long-term impact the GMO products may have on consumers.

I just finished reading a headline in our local newspaper: "Student Dies After Seven Days in a Coma." It seems he ingested some peanut butter and had an allergic reaction. He drove himself to the hospital and passed out before making it inside. Apparently, he had been allergic to peanuts all of his life. I think we are looking at this all wrong. We should be looking at the pesticides growing in our crops, and see if that is where the connection lies. Pesticides are a chemical poison for heaven's sake! We should not be having fatal reactions from our foods. No one should have to live like that.

That's why it's a good idea to sign petitions to demand that GMO food be labeled GMO. We're standing at the crossroads of an industry that's not protecting our health. We must step up to the plate (pun intended). Safeguard your health by displaying a healthy amount of skepticism and asking lots of questions when you shop for groceries, and whenever someone in a white jacket tries to convince you to take too many pills.

8

DON'T GIVE UP!

I was talking to a colleague about this book and I realized some of the issues discussed did not include what I am about to say now. It is about my baby brothers – the identical twins. You see, they both suffered from schizophrenia. It started at the tender young age of eight. One of the twins had a breakdown and had to be hospitalized. He was then moved to a children's center in the state. The other twin suffered the same fate around the age of twelve. They were in a state mental institution as adults, and went on to live independently in supervised homes – at least one twin did.

In 1971, twin #1 died at the age of 18, and I started having panic attacks. I'm pretty sure his death is what pushed me over the edge. I was at the hospital when he was admitted. I saw the blood bags that caused me to become faint and nauseous. Hospital personnel, seeing my distress, took me out of the room, sat me down, and made me bend over. They put my head between my knees and asked me to breathe, while they opened the doors to let in more air. I soon recovered physically, but not mentally. It was horrifying for me to see what he had to go through—that this mental disorder could cause him to hallucinate to the point of dying.

I do remember twin #2. Between twin #1's death and the funeral, he woke up with a patch of grey at the top front of his hairline. It seemed to me that his hair turned white overnight! So, just imagine what his grief must have been like. Twins are inseparable. Identical twins? I cannot fathom his feelings. I think I took the death the hardest. I was in despair. It took some comforting words from a friend to bring me some measure of peace. She said, "God has to have some good people on his side." That statement was the only thing that calmed me down and got me through it. I can only imagine what my mother must have been experiencing.

When something happens in an immediate family, it causes trauma for the whole family. Being the eldest, I had to deal with the fact that my mother had shut down. It was all too much for her. I had to be the strong person and that proved to be too much for me as well. So, dealing with death and dealing with separation and divorce at the same time had a devastating effect on my physical and mental wellbeing.

This was the second death in our family. The first was my oldest brother, killed while serving his country. I never realized that I was still grieving until recently. I got depressed every Memorial Day Holiday for the last several years. I can't even say that he was killed in action because it turned out to be an accident. The term used is "friendly fire." In his case, it was pilot error. And they never even told us the cause until I started an investigation through my state representative. So, I never had closure, and when something is not resolved, it can have a detrimental effect on your mental and physical health over many years. At least that is what happened to me.

I remember being awake that night my mother got the dreaded knock at our door, and two officers stood outside. She screamed and ran to the back of the house where my sister and I slept. She was told he was missing in action. Everything was a blur after that, and the funeral was planned and executed with two marines standing on guard at our home. There was no body, only a dog tag. No one can ever know the depth of chaos that went on in my family, and in me, with that revelation. I started sleepwalking. I became a nervous wreck, and my world just changed.

At the funeral, my mother took the flag that was presented to her while they played "Taps." She held her head up and didn't shed a tear. It was the saddest moment of my life. I can only speak about my personal experience in trying to cope with this tragedy. My sister and I cried our eyes out that day.

Between these deaths and my failed marriage, I thought my world as I knew it was over. I lost my focus in life. But, I forgot that I am my mother's daughter. I came back fighting and I won!

9

TRIUMPH AND VICTORY!

I feel like I have been reborn. Seriously, ever since I conquered the health crises that had derailed me for years, I feel as if I have blossomed into a sparkling and exciting wife, mother, and career woman. The old me was a tired and frazzled shell of what I am. But the woman who has now emerged is radiant, energetic, and ready to take on the world.

I took control and I have reversed my bone loss and I am thrilled to report that I have my life back. It has been a 14-year journey, but people tell me I am looking younger and looking well.

I feel attractive again! What's more, I'm basking in flattery and admiration. Everywhere I go, folks come up to me and tell me how gorgeous my hair is, and how well I look. Now, I usually get compliments, instead of the dreaded question, "Are you OK?" It feels good to be receiving positive feedback. I especially like the fact that much of that feedback is directed towards my hair. People had occasionally praised my hair in the past, but I don't think anyone had ever called it "gorgeous."

These days, comments on my glowing appearance and health are commonplace. At first, I was stunned by these out-of-the-blue compliments about the luster and bounce of my hair. Our hair is a reflection of the state of our health. I'm glad that people are validating the results of all my efforts to regain my wellbeing. All these people couldn't be wrong, could they? Interestingly enough, most of my admirers are saying the exact same thing: "Your hair is beautiful!" It's uncanny. I must admit, it's been wonderful getting this kind of attention at my age because, believe me, it is no picnic being sick and worn out. It's just the pits. I remember posing for a picture back then, looking at it and thinking how matronly and old I looked. Some people might find this amusing, but this was serious business to me. It's more than just vanity. Most of my life, I'd been tiny with a beautiful figure… and there I was, watching in horror as all of my attributes slipped away. I couldn't believe it!

Thank God, that crazy chapter in my life is over!

CRAZY! HOT! and LIVING ON THE EDGE!

I'm finished with canes, and I'm getting less "mam" greetings, and more smiles and nods. Of course, I'm extremely glad to be healthy again, but looking good is an added bonus. I never looked my age anyway, so why should I start catching up to it now?

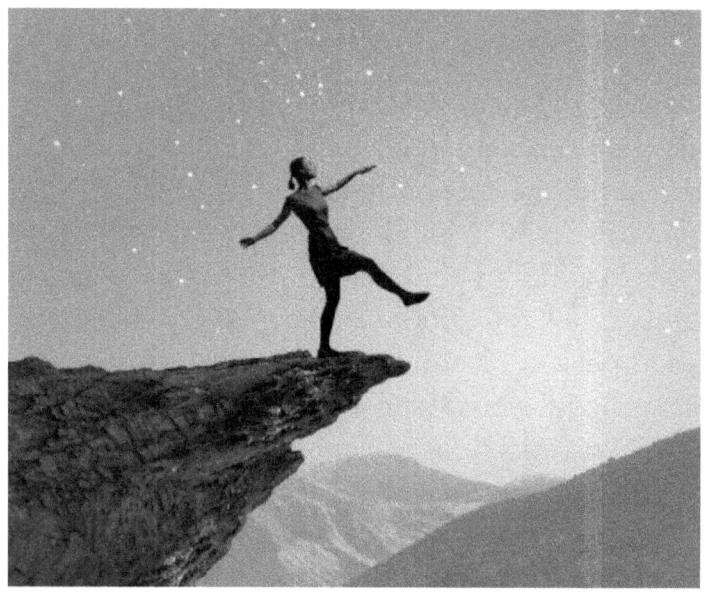

So, what do I do to maintain my vigor and happiness?

I have a conventional doctor and an alternative doctor, and I work with both of them. I regard natural medicine as complementary medicine. Some people don't think holistic practices are compatible with traditional medicine. However, they are wrong! When given a chance, the two can fit together quite well.

For instance, if you must take a drug or have surgery, the knowledge you acquire can help you make better choices. A holistic doctor or herbalist can point out the juices, fruits, herbs and veggies that will help ward off side effects and assist your body as you recover.

I have a friend who was diagnosed with lung cancer and she is taking a chemo pill which helps to keep the cancer at bay; and she's incorporating supplements and herbs to complement what she is doing. A natural diet and vitamins promote healing, and offers the nutritional boost her body needs. She spent three weeks at an alternative healing and detox facility out of San Diego, TX. She ate wheat grass to detox, and lots of raw, uncooked vegetables. I am gratified to know that she found some help for her affliction. She is energetic and not sick at all while fighting cancer. She is able to travel and do pretty much what she wants.

The key is to know when to go natural, when to heed conventional advice, and when to blend the two. I listen to my heart and make sure I'm giving my body, mind, and spirit, all the love, rest, attention and natural antidotes needed.

My daily routine goes something like this:

- Rise - 9:00 am. Breakfast.

- Stretch Exercises.
- Lunch – 1:00/2:00 pm.
- Read or meditate.
- Writing or editing.
- Breathing exercises and reminders to stay centered.
- Dinner with husband - 5:30/6:00 pm.
- Possibly a few phone conversations with friends (Positive phone calls only).
- Relax and enjoy comedic or inspirational TV programs.
- Pray (This is a must!).
- Gratitude (I try to keep a gratitude journal listing all the things I'm thankful for.).
- A daily dose of laughter (It's an important addition to your medicine chest of natural cures).

This is the regimen I try to stick to (laughter and all). I work at it all the time. Sometimes I watch a political program and get upset. So, I have to learn to stay away from those as much as possible.

I try to select shows that put me in a good mood. Seriously, the endorphins (sedative-like chemicals produced by the brain) created by laughter, are a good prescription for whatever is ailing you. In fact, a medical doctor by the name of Norman Cousins, author of the book, "Anatomy of an Illness" actually cured himself of cancer by renting funny movies and laughing all day long for months. Later, he coined the term "Laughter Therapy" and began incorporating it as a treatment for his patients.

How about that? Who knew that something as simple as laughing could help ease our woes? But when you think about it for a minute, it makes a lot of sense. Everything we do, from crying to smiling, from singing to screaming, serves a purpose. Our bodies are uniquely designed to self-heal, and sometimes it's as simple as tapping into our inner child spirit and unleashing a little humor.

So, I fill my day with ripples of laughter. In other words, I put joy on my schedule. I plan to have a good time by looking for activities that inspire me and fill me with peace. At times, I even shake my itinerary up a bit by going on a day-long or three-day retreat with my church or on a fun-filled vacation with my husband. Throw in a little bit of the Wendy Williams Show for good measure. It makes me laugh a lot!

Vacations, by the way, are another diversion that can be credited for keeping people healthy. If you can't afford one, find an easy and inexpensive outlet. Examples include: ballroom dance classes, dinner and a movie, a nice stroll along the river, an early evening bike ride (fun at any age), or a get together with friends at a juice bar that makes delicious smoothies (the healthy ones made with real fruit and veggies). You might even conquer a fear and try something you've never tried before – like rock climbing, taking a Zumba class, going to a wine tasting class, or joining Toastmasters and giving a speech. Toastmasters is an interesting group because everyone there is testing out their public speaking skills. I used to attend Toastmasters once a week before work. It was conveniently located right inside the Detroit Free Press building where I was employed. It was fascinating and challenging to me—trying to conquer my personal fear of speaking.

Supposedly, it's in the top 10 list of personal human fears. If you try Toastmasters, you might beat this fear, or not. Either way, you'd have fun laughing at and congratulating yourself. You'll get an adrenalin rush, and the feeling of confidence that comes from trying something new.

While not in the best of health, I managed to work on a campaign to help rescue a local train station from neglect and ruin. I jumped in the midst of the chaos, and busily did all I could to pull it off. When I say Action, Cameras, Lights, I mean that literally. I relied on city services and solicited assistance from the city's movers and shakers, and the Citizen's District Council in Corktown. I did all this while taking college courses; this project was an "Applied Research Project" and I earned an A.I even ended up on the evening news. The train station project was the lead story for the night, and everyone involved was jockeying for their 15 minutes of fame. I wasn't seeking fame, but I was the one who created it so I was interviewed.

At the time, I had gotten laid off from my job as a Classified Sales Representative for the "Detroit Free Press" and had a lot of pent up anger that manifested itself in this project. All my frustrations made me more creative. I didn't know I had it in me. As president of the New Friends of the Michigan Central Depot, I created a newsletter called "On Track" and wrote an article about what inspired me to save our train station. The Detroit Free Press was impressed and I was featured in the same paper that had laid me off. What an irony! And all the while, my health was in jeopardy.

People didn't even know I was suffering. I didn't know I was descending into a crisis of health either. I didn't sit back – I jumped out there and kept looking for exciting new possibilities, and new opportunities to distract me and help clear my head of the mental cobwebs and other frustrations that often block our inner peace.

Whatever you choose, remember there's nothing like activity and a little rest and relaxation to help you decompress and get your mind and spirit focused. In fact, there's an old saying that goes, "Free your mind and your body will follow." There's another saying that's even more popular: "You're too blessed to be stressed."

Well, they might be clichés, but they're true. When you're happy, the cells in your body are rejoicing right along with you. When you're calm, you're literally taking a "chill pill," and your body's cells are responding accordingly. In my case, my immune system has never been better. I still get allergic reactions to drugs, so my goal is to keep them few and far between.

I hate to sound like I'm always knocking the medical establishment, but I came away with a bad taste in my mouth because they didn't know what to do with me. As a result, they preferred to not deal with me at all. After being forced to take control of my health, I began keeping track of all of my medical records, and studying the history of what I endured and what I was prescribed.

This helps me measure what works for me and what doesn't. And it assists me if I'm in a situation where drugs can't be avoided. I still suffer with drug side-affects if I have to take them. Nowadays, the only time that happens is when I go to the dentist with a toothache, an abscess in a tooth, or some sort of surgery. When you're dealing with that kind of pain, trust me, you won't be able to resist some type of painkiller. But I dread it because when it comes to drugs, I still don't trust them. After one dental visit, I suffered a horrible reaction to Acetaminophen – Codeine #3. And so I scratched that one off my list. Actually, I made a list of drugs that I have had a reaction to, and hand them out whenever I meet a doctor I've never seen before, especially my new dentist and dental specialists.

It took a while for me to find the right balance between my conventional doctor and my alternative doctor, but it can be done. Now, I have them both working with me. It wasn't easy because doctors are so educated that you can't speak up against their beliefs. You have to tread carefully so as not to trample on their egos. It's a balancing act for sure. I better be careful in my judgment of doctors because I have one now who works well with me. The services he provides are helping so much that I don't feel the need to see him all the time. Working with his assistant is just fine with me. Before, I used to panic whenever I couldn't see the actual doctor.

That's not the case now. I am comfortable because I know what's happening with my body, and I know what works and what I need to avoid. It's a scary thought, knowing that you have to take precautionary steps to protect yourself from a bad drug reaction or, heaven forbid, the side effects of major or minor surgery. I pray every time, but of late, I have not been sick enough to entertain that thought. The key for me is to stay well. Now that my immune system is up and

I am not prone to getting sick, not a day goes by that I don't celebrate my healthy, youthful body and spirit. I'm so thankful that I was led down the right path to wellness. I don't think I would be here if I had not found some alternative solutions.

But the journey continues. In 2014, I saw my regular doctor for a checkup. I was asked to undergo a Dexa Scan -- a bone density scan of my hip area. I made a follow-up visit with the doctor to discuss the results. Turns out, I have some bone loss progression in my spine and hips. My doctor recommended that I take Fosomax. I read up on the drug and was horrified at the side-effects. With my history of drug interaction problems, I opted out of his suggestion. I told him I would consult with my alternative specialist, Dr. Pamela Smith, M.D., MPH. She is a medical doctor with a master's in public health.

I left his office visibly shaken. I was not expecting to hear that kind of news.

I have been experiencing some unusual stomach upsets after ingesting hormone pills and multivitamins, starting in the morning. This went on for a couple of years before I told the doctor about my suffering, and being informed that I should not be feeling that way. I started writing down what I was doing and narrowed down the cause. I was ingesting the hormone pills without food, which was not the right way to do it.

If you are suffering from diarrhea and constipation, how can you nourish your body adequately? That might explain the bone loss. But I'm just speculating here. I do that a lot.

It also means that I will have to get back to my health regimen, including more exercise. I have slacked off a little bit. It's not easy, but it's better than the alternative. I will go back to my juicing regimen. I haven't juiced for quite some time.

See! There is a solution for everything that ails you.

Dr. Smith has given me a supplement that I am now taking in place of Fosomax. She has also ramped up my vitamin D intake. I don't want to name the supplements because what works for me may not work for someone else, and I wouldn't want to be responsible or be accused of making unauthorized medical recommendations. The point is to help you to understand that there are choices out there and I encourage you to take advantage of them.

Did you know that there is an organic juice concoction for bone health? Well, there is. And I'm going to try it. I'm going to gently remind myself that I cannot abandon the practices that got me where I am today. This advice applies to everyone. Remain vigilant and do not slack off of these programs or you might find some of your health issues reoccurring. Consistency is important.

Here is the recipe for your bones. It was out of the menu planner that came with my juicer:

HEALTHY BONE TONIC
Supplies calcium for maintenance of healthy bones

Ingredients:

6 carrots

4 kale leaves

4 sprigs parsley

½ apple

Please use organic veggies only.

Remember, knowledge is power! I challenge each and every individual reading this book to find it before it is too late. Take a page from my story.

10

HOW TO MAINTAIN YOUR RECORDS

You have to do some extra work in order to keep up with your health, like keeping records of your medical history. Keep track of your past lab tests on a regular basis, like a colonoscopy or breast exam. You can lose track of when you need to go again, especially if you are prone to changing doctors like I was. Don't count on your doctor to keep track, although with computers, they do seem to be doing a better job.

Organization is the key to good health. Here are a few tips for getting your records in shape:

1. Save the documentation from your doctor's visit, such as prescriptions, lab results, instructions, etc. Put them in a big envelope. I

had to track down old surgical records by visiting the hospital and asking for them. Luckily, I got them and I filed them properly after that.

2. Write down any medications that affect you adversely. I had to go back and find records, and rely on memory because I did not write anything down. I keep my allergies and drug reactions on an index card now. When you need the information, having a file will come in handy.

3. Write down any and everything that you're having problems with. A journal will help you keep important health concerns within reach, if you need to refer back to them.

4. Make a list of the drugs you're are taking, and your adverse reactions to them, if any, so that you can inform your brand new doctor, who doesn't know you yet. I handed out a sheet to my doctor, dentist, and dental specialist. I was having some dental work done and the dentist needed to be aware of the drugs I have problems with.

When I told Dr. Smith about the trouble I was having with the side-effects of penicillin, she asked me if I was taking the enzyme supplement she recommended. I said no. I had forgotten about it. So I re-ordered it, and it helped me get through the stomach problems associated with penicillin.

You must pay attention and write down whatever your conventional or alternative doctor (if you have one) recommends, so you can keep up with his/her instructions. I had a problem with this, but got it under control. Never depend on anyone but yourself to keep up with the drugs, vitamins or supplements that you're taking. The doctor can't do it all and we shouldn't want them to. What if something were to happen to that doctor? You would be "up a creek" trying to carry on without him/her around. Oh sure, they keep records, but not as accurate as your records can be. You're the one who's taking them and would know better. Besides, asking for your records cost money. I had a doctor that wouldn't release my records to my current doctor. There doesn't seem to be any honor between medical practitioners. Everything is business. That incident taught me a valuable lesson. Keep a journal. You can go back to it for any information needed. Throw your yearly journal into that big brown envelope as well when you're done with it.

Do whatever works for you… but do it. These days, what works might not be mainstream and that's okay. As you focus on maintaining records, also make a list of new and different alternative health modalities that you have explored or hope to explore.

Some of the more obscure modalities include:

Reflexology – A natural healing practice that involves applying pressure to specific points in the ears, hands, and at the bottom of the feet. These pressure points correspond to specific organs and glands in the body.

Iridology – An alternative medicine technique which claims that patterns, colors, and other characteristics of the iris can be examined to gather information about a patient's systemic health.

Acupuncture – Acupuncture is one of the main forms of treatment in traditional Chinese medicine. It involves the use of sharp, thin needles that are inserted in the body at very specific points.

Inversion table – If you have back, neck or other physical pain, an inversion table can provide therapy. The table inverts the body and allows you to hang upside down. It's great for the spine, and some people believe that it helps our body defy gravity and delays the aging process.

Tai Chi – A slow moving exercise based on an ancient Chinese tradition of using gentle body movements to harness the flow of positive energy. Benefits include increased flexibility, enhanced immune system, and a decrease in joint pain.

Reiki Healing – This is an unusual technique that typically involves lying on a table while a healer directs your energy without touching you. The healer moves his or her hands in a motion that is said to help relieve pain and anxiety.

Check out these techniques and if any of them resonate with you, add them to your list. It's also a good idea to write down your own personal tried-and-true antidotes – ideas that no one may have considered but you.

For example, if you have an allergic reaction to something, and you noticed that opening a window or drinking lots of fluids helps you get through the episode, then make a note of that. In other words, you might have personal ways of coping that are unique to you.

Keep a record of whatever you do – no matter how absurd it may seem. I have a friend who swears that her headaches go away whenever she hears soft music. Another friend used to exercise during her menstrual cycle because she said it helped with her cramps. Others with cramps insist that they can't exercise at all during that time of the month.

In some cases, one person will swear that a daily one-mile run is all they need to stay focused and in good health. Still others insist that a weekly massage or a nightly soak in a Jacuzzi positively impacts their health. Basically, I'm advising you to do what works for you, and write it down so that you'll remember to try it again when the need arises. I'm also suggesting that you read as much as you can in order to stay on top of what's happening in the food and drug industry. In addition, sign petitions. This might sound like a minor activity or something that can't possibly solve the problem. However, it can and does make a difference.

I belong to a company called Credo Mobile that sends out petitions which help ordinary individuals impact what's going on in our environment, our food supply, and holding our politicians accountable when necessary. When you sign one of their petitions, you become an activist who is making his/her voice heard. These petitions urge the FDA to keep Genetically Modified (GMO) salmon out of the United States. They also push for limits and labels on GMO produce.

We have to protect our right to pursue good health. This includes what we eat, the drugs we are given, organic food choices, and natural supplements to good health. We need the choices. Don't let those be taken away. There are forces out there trying to do just that! It's really scary and you can't afford not to be informed. It's never too late to start, but always remember... nothing is ever easy.

Consider this manual your personal resource. Follow it and learn what you can from someone who was once "crazy, hot, and living on the edge" and emerged to not only talk about it, but to help lead the way!

Summary

WHAT YOU CAN DO!

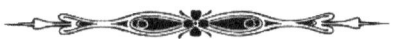

Here are some common sense things you can do to help yourself and your family overcome many afflictions.

- Start a diary or journal of everything going on with you, and how you are feeling. Write down what you are eating, and what drugs you're taking.
- Cleanse your colon. You don't need a doctor's permission to do that. Google "Colonics" to find a center in your area. Mine is The Detroit Wholistic Center, run by Jesse Brown, N.D., located on Grand River and Burt Road, Detroit.
- Get some sort of probiotics (digestive enzymes) back into your gut. There are health aids at the health stores if you don't have a doctor who can prescribe something. Many doctors are learning more and are willing to listen to their patients.
- Find an alternative doctor to work with you, who fits your specific needs. Start learning about your symptoms. I found the *Centers for Healthy Living and*

Longevity headed by Dr. Pamela Smith to help me with my specific issues. Visit this site for a referral: http://www.centerforpersonalizedmedicine.com/

- If you can't afford to see doctors, then start a juicing regimen. You can buy a juicer with recipes and instructions included. Always use organic fruits and vegetables. Just remember that pesticides are in conventional fruits and vegetables, and you will get ill if you don't watch what you're putting in your juicer and into your body. Apples are notorious for pesticides. Avoid them! Invest in a juicer or power blender, and/or food processor. Whatever works for you, do it! Juicing and power-blending works for me.
- For body cleansing and physical health therapy, if you can afford it, attend a resort or spa. Make sure they have good reviews.
- Again, eat or drink your vegetables. I cannot stress this enough. You will be amazed at the results. Vegetables are nature's miracle workers.
- I once suffered with shortness of breath. That is the beginning stages of heart disease. Getting on a hormone therapy regimen cleared all of that up. I was pleasantly surprised by that benefit. Now, I can climb the stairs without being out of breath. But make sure that before you start treating any symptom, you know what is wrong with you. Don't self-diagnose.

- Digestive disorders can be cured in the early stages, and you don't need drugs or surgery to do it. I had to stop taking antibiotics. Eliminating all drugs was my solution, since I suffered from side effects big time. Cabbage juice is a natural cure for diverticulitis. For a bladder infection, use organic cranberry juice.
- For beautiful skin and gorgeous hair – just juice. That's all your fruits and veggies in a glass. You will see immediate results, I promise.
- Shop at places like Whole Foods. They are all across the country, including Detroit and its suburbs. I shop at Natural Food Patch in Ferndale, MI. Be proactive in knowing which foods are beneficial to your health.
- See a conventional doctor on a regular basis, and take control of your health in the meantime by seeking out the advice of herbalists and other holistic specialists.
- If you have a significant other, don't forget to take care of him/her too. If you are eating right, your spouse also eats right.
- Get on a multivitamin regimen. Make sure there are no synthetic ingredients in the capsules. Go to a health store and read labels. Whole food vitamins like New Chapter are best, because your body recognizes them as real food.
- Eliminate sugar. It's the number one cause of bad health.

- Exercise. I do stretches and that works for me.
- Drink herbal teas. I recommend chamomile, ginger, and licorice. Ginger and licorice soothe the digestive system.
- Only buy foods labeled non-GMO.
- Every now and then, add raw foods to your diet. Snack on raw carrots, celery, and other veggies. Of course, include raw fruit.
- Eat only wild-caught fish. Farm-raised fish swims around in an environment that can be compared to a cesspool. If you must do farm raised, make sure the label indicates that it was farm-raised responsibly, meaning that the conditions were clean, and the fish are free of antibiotics.
- When possible, drink alkaline or purified water. I have a reverse osmosis system installed in my home.
- Try to fit Therapeutic Massages into your routine. Once a month is ideal, but it also helps if you only get one every three to six months. Massages do wonders for stress. Besides soothing aching muscles, they also help release toxins from the body.

Appendix

TERMS YOU SHOULD KNOW

Bio-Identical Hormone Therapy – Natural Hormone Replacement Therapy that's close to human hormones

Colon Cleanse – A cleansing process that uses water to draw waste from your body in a controlled environment.

Diverticulosis – A disease caused by lack of fiber in diet. Pockets are formed in the colon and food becomes trapped, causing infection with severe pain.

Digestive Enzymes – Tablets containing friendly bacteria that is necessary for good digestion. Information can be found on the internet.

Ear Wax Buildup – Eliminate dairy products from the diet and this will go away.

Food & Fragrance Allergies – A bad reaction to processed foods and some vegetables. Intolerance or bad reaction to cleaning sprays, perfumes, and chemicals.

Heart Disease – If the blood supply to the heart muscle is cut off, a heart attack can result. Cells in the heart muscles do not receive enough oxygen and begin to die. The more time that passes without treatment to restore blood flow, the greater the damage to the heart.

Hot Flashes - Symptoms associated with Hormone imbalance or depletion.

Hysterectomy – Surgical procedure to remove reproductive organs.

Impacted Bowels – Waste in the bowels that cannot empty itself; severe constipation. Caused by too much fast food, and no fiber in the diet.

Irritable Bowel Syndrome (IBS) - Not sure if dairy products cause it, or if IBS causes the lactose intolerance, but it's a catch 22. Dairy is believed to be the culprit, and definitely the western diet.

Menopause – Lack of female hormones to regulate the body. Occurs when menstruation ceases for a period of one year.

Menstruation – Blood flow from the uterus to prepare for conception. The monthly process starts during puberty in young girls.

Migraines – Severe head pain with an aura present in the line of vision. Try Colonics and eliminate dairy products. Also, try to reduce the stress in your life.

Osteoporosis – Thinning of bones, causing loss of bone density.

Panic Attacks – Symptoms include shortness of breath, tightening of the chest, fainting, rapid heartbeat, and a feeling of impending doom.

Hyperventilation Syndrome -- A respiratory disorder, psychologically or physiologically based, which involves breathing too deeply or too rapidly (hyperventilation). Many people with panic disorder will experience HVS.

Acknowledgement

I want to acknowledge the President of *Rave Reviews Book Club*, whose encouragement helped me to see that the story needed to be told.

I want to thank my dear and wonderful friend, Mamie Smith, who supports me in all my endeavors.

Thank you, Lolita, for the beautiful artwork. You captured exactly what I was looking for. What a great gift you have.

Thank you, Herb Metoyer, for helping me get this book to the finish line. Your expertise was very much appreciated and needed. You left us much too soon.

Thanks to everyone who came in contact with me throughout this process, including my wonderful support group at Rave Reviews Book Club. I appreciate all of you for being supporters and good critics.

About the Author

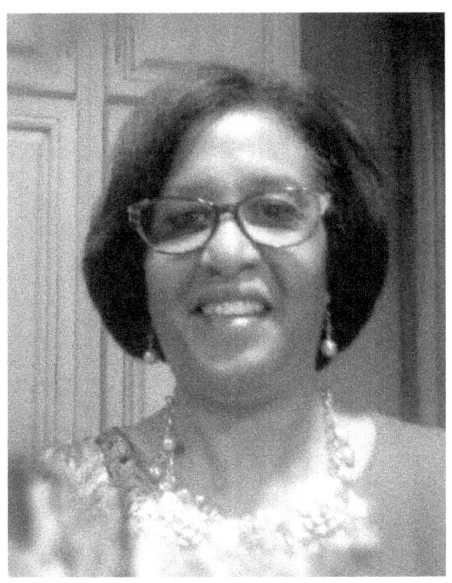

Shirley Harris-Slaughter's first book highlights her passion for history which led to her first published work, *Our Lady of Victory, the Saga of an African American Catholic Community.* But she wouldn't have been able to write that book had she not had the presence of mind to conquer the health crisis she found herself in. She is an advocate for natural health and healing. Any problem she had to face she found her way out of, through sheer determination and a miracle.

This led to her second book, CRAZY! HOT! AND LIVING ON THE EDGE!!

Shirley saw a void that needed to be filled, and so she decided to share her experience.

She has been active in her community by supporting candidates for elected office. She served on the Oak Park School Board. She is an advocate for children, and mentored four freshmen girls in the Winning Futures program. Shirley is an active member in her church and she belongs to the Rave Reviews (Virtual) Book Club. She married her best friend, Langston, and they share a blended family.

"We are as different as night and day, and yet we are so much alike in many ways. We made it through thirty-two years!"

Shirley Harris-Slaughter is available for book events and speaking engagements.

sharrislaughter@gmail.com